Did I Make Par?

By Ken Hines

Copyright

ISBN-978-0-9723895-1-8

Contents

Chapter One

Charlie was alive and breathing, but temporarily brain-dead. He didn't remember walking up to the eighteenth green, removing the ball from the cup, shaking hands with his playing partner, walking off the green and into the scorer's tent to sign his scorecard, or anything else for that matter. He was not even aware of hearing the roar of the crowd. Charlie was simply in a deep and confusing fog as he made his way out of the scorer's tent and through the crowd. He absent-mindedly signed scorecards, caps or anything someone put in front of him.

Abe, his caddie, saw Charlie as soon as he walked out of the tent and began the trek through the crowd of golfing fans. Abe shrugged his shoulders and dove into the crowd to rescue Charlie. "Hey, man. Let's get out of here," Abe said quite loudly when he reached his golfer.

Charlie looked at Abe and muttered. "Okay."

As the two made their way through the last of the crowd and reached the semi safe area of the player's parking lot, Abe spoke first. "Hey Charlie, it wasn't that bad. Not everyone can say they blew fifty-thousand dollars and a guaranteed return to the next US Open on the last hole, huh?"

Charlie looked at his caddie like a deer looking into the headlights of a sixteen wheeler bearing down at seventy miles per hour on the interstate. "Yeah, I guess so," replied Charlie.

There was a few seconds of silence from both of them. Charlie finally came around, touched Abe on the shoulder and said, "Abe, I'm sorry. I guess I really screwed the pooch today, huh?"

"Hey, don't sweat it man. You still came in tied for fourteenth. That has to be good for a couple of thousand. Shit… having a guaranteed invite back to the tournament next year is no big thing anyway. We can always qualify again," Abe added.

Charlie looked at Abe and tried to smile but it looked like he just walked out of the dentist office with a mouth full of Novocain. One side of his mouth went slightly up but the other side was just not responding.

Abe looked at his friend and said, "That is what I call a smile of happiness, my friend. Hell, the ball you ended up with on the 18th today had a better smile on it."

Charlie heard that wise-crack and smiled. It was almost a genuine, broad smile. "We gave them their money's worth though, didn't we?"

"You can say that again," Abe said.

"Fuck it, Abe. Let's get out of here and go get a beer."

"Now you're talking. Let's go. The beer here costs too damn much and the atmosphere sucks," replied Abe.

The two were walking to Charlie's beat up Chrysler when Diane walked up from the side.

"Boy, you two were something to watch today," she said.

Charlie smiled really big this time and watched Diane walk the rest of the way up to them. "Well, we had a good time. Just wish I could remember what we did on the last hole," he added with a bit of humor.

Diane laughed out loud.

Charlie stuck out his hand, which was quickly grabbed by Diane.

"Thanks," Charlie said softly. "I expected you to head the other way after I screwed up the last hole. I'm really glad you're here right now."

"My pleasure," Diane replied just as softly.

Abe walked ahead and had the clubs in the car and grabbed Charlie's regular shoes out of the trunk and handed them to Charlie. Charlie took the shoes and was about to change them when he suddenly stopped and looked at Diane. "You wouldn't want to spend the rest of your life with a dumb, beaten up golf pro, would you?" he asked.

Without hesitating one little bit, she responded, "Sure I would, if he's already beaten up, it saves me from having to do it myself."

Charlie was stunned and for the moment forgot about changing his shoes. He grabbed Diane, hugged her and lifted her up off her feet. "This is much better than winning the Open," he added.

The two were still embraced with Abe watching silently when two men walked up. Charlie thought he recognized one of the men but wasn't sure. He set Diane back on her feet and turned toward the two men walking up.

"Don't tell me I signed the wrong card," Charlie said to the men thinking they were with the tournament.

"No, you didn't sign the wrong card. We just wanted to catch you before you left. Not sure if you would be interested in it but we have a possible proposition for you, Charlie," the taller gentleman said.

Charlie smiled cautiously. "That depends on what the proposition is," he added.

"Charlie, we are from San Antonio and I'm one of the members of the Pecan Valley Country Club. My name is

Harry Todd and this gentleman is Ned Woolfolk. Ned is the manager of our club and would like to talk to you about something."

Charlie turned toward Ned. "I know, I know. You guys want the ball that I finished up with. I threw it into the stands. I guess I can't give you that one." Charlie reached into his bag and pulled out a beat up Titleist. He handed the ball toward Ned. "You can put that on the wall in your pro shop," he added.

Ned looked somewhat surprised by Charlie's action. "No, we don't want the ball," he said pausing a bit. "That is, unless the owner of the ball comes with it."

Charlie looked totally surprised before realizing that they probably wanted him to give a clinic at the club. "Okay, you want me to drop by your club and give a demonstration on how to not finish a professional golf tournament?" he asked.

"No, Charlie, that's not it either," Ned responded. "Harry and I have watched you for the last four days. You've got a great golf game and more importantly, everyone seems to really like you. You had twenty thousand golfers routing for you today and that really says something. We watched the crowd when you walked off the 18th green and almost everyone wanted to get close to you. I think you would be the perfect fit to be the head golf pro at Pecan Valley. Your play during this tournament shows that you have the game needed and the way you handled the pressure says a lot about your character. You are someone that knows what he wants and then goes for it and that's exactly what we need. Pecan Valley has been struggling for members lately and we both think that you would be the person to take charge of our club in San Antonio and bring our membership up. How does that sound?"

At first, Charlie was speechless. He turned toward Diane and looked at her.

8

She smiled and, eyes wide open, formed an inquisitive look on her face.

Charlie again looked at Ned. "Well, that sounds very interesting. Of course, I'll have to discuss it with my wife… or I should say future wife. It so happens that just before you two guys walked up, I sort of proposed to this beautiful lady here and I think she accepted."

Harry was the first to respond, "Charlie, that's super. I was wondering why she was hugging you. Let me be the first to congratulate both of you. Hell, you can have your wedding at the club."

"Harry, you're going too fast," Ned responded. "Let's let these two discuss our proposal and they can get back to us".

Charlie looked at Diane and she nodded a small approval. Charlie nodded back to Diane.

"Ned, I've worked with Abe for several years and I'd like to be sure he has a spot there too. Abe is the only person that I know who can get grass to grow in Lubbock. We only have a small, nine-hole track but our greens were as good as the greens for this year's Open. Hell, if I say so myself, our greens are better. I don't know who you have as the superintendent but Abe could really help him," Charlie responded.

Everyone looked at Abe for a response. He just shrugged his shoulders and replied, "Hell, this is the strangest day of my life. My pro just lost the Open, got engaged and has been offered a job in San Antonio. What the hell, if it's Okay with Charlie, it's Okay with me. Count me in too."

"Gentlemen, you just got yourself a golf professional," Charlie said. "When do you want us to start?"

"Well, there's no big rush. Take your time and let's say you drop by sometime towards the end of the week. How does,

Thursday around twelve sound? We can have lunch while we go over the details of the job. If you like the club and the offer, we've got a deal."

"Okay, we will be there Thursday," Charlie answered smiling. "We were just getting ready to head down to the nearest bar and have a beer or two. You guys want to come along?"

"No, but thanks for the offer," replied Ned. "Harry and I need to wrap up a couple of things here and then head back to San Antonio."

The two men walked back toward the clubhouse and Charlie looked at Diane and smiled. "Damn, that was a big surprise, huh?"

"Yes it was," she replied. "You have a way about you Charlie. I hope I can figure it out one day."

"Good luck on that, Diane," said Abe. "I've known the son-of-a-bitch for ten years now and I don't know how this shit happens. Let's go get a beer and I'll tell you some more stories about Charlie."

The three stopped at the first watering hole they came to and Charlie ordered three Long Necks. Holding up the first beer, Charlie touched bottles with Diane and then Abe. "Here's to one of the strangest days in my life. I blew the lead at the US Open on the last hole. I got engaged to the most beautiful woman in the world. I landed a great head professional job at a super club and also got a great job for my best friend."

"I'll drink to that," Diane added.

"Me too," replied Abe.

They drank quite a few beers before checking into the nearest motel.

Charlie woke up the next morning and couldn't believe his eyes. He had the most beautiful woman in the world lying next to him and studying his face intently.

"Good morning beautiful," Charlie said in a whisper. "I was hoping you'd still be here in the morning."

Diane smiled as she kept eye contact and continued to study Charlie's face. "I thought about it but I know my life would really suck without having you in it. So, I'm still here and plan to be looking at your eyes in the morning for the rest of my life."

Charlie didn't say anything but kissed her gently on the lips.

Diane started to say something but the sudden snoring noise from the other bed in the room got her attention first. It was Abe who made the noise but it also caused him to awaken.

Abe slowly opened his eyes before rolling over in bed. He had quite a few beers the previous evening and wasn't thinking very clearly yet. He looked over at the other bed and could barely make out the back of a strange woman facing away from him. "God-damn, Charlie. Who did you pick up last night?" he asked.

Diane laughed out loud. Holding the sheet against her breasts, she turned around and looked at Abe. "Good morning," she said.

Abe was surprised but the events of yesterday afternoon slowly began to come around. "Oh, shit, it's you Diane. I thought that you would have come to your senses and book out of here in the middle of the night."

"I'm still here. However, in the future, I think that you will be getting your own room," she said. "It's not that I'm shy but your snoring shook the walls last night."

11

Charlie looked over Diane's shoulder and peered at Abe. "Good morning, amigo," he said with a huge smile on his face. "She's still here. That's got to be a first, huh."

"Yeah," replied Abe. "I remember that time in Amarillo when we went out after you won that tournament. We both picked up these two…"

Abe was cut off by Diane. "Okay, Abe. Let's not compare me to ladies from the past. I'm here and will be here for some time to come. I don't want to hear about Charlie's other exploits… or yours for that matter."

"Oh, Okay," said Abe.

"Abe, pull the covers over your head. I'm going to get up and take a shower. We need to head to San Antonio today so I can introduce Charlie to my parents. That will be interesting but I need to be ready. You and Charlie here will also need to clean up too," she added. "Now cover up and I'll get up."

Abe didn't say anything but quickly pulled the covers over his head.

Diane turned back to Charlie and gave him a good, long kiss. "Give me about ten minutes and I'll be out of the shower."

She got out of the bed and quickly got her clothes and stepped into the bathroom, closing the door.

The noise from the shower was Abe's signal to pull the covers down from over his head. He turned toward Charlie who was looking at him already. "Man, are you sure you want to do this?" Abe asked.

"This is the only girl I've ever wanted to have in my bed in the morning. Hell, you've known me for over ten years and have you ever have known me to have a woman in my bed in the morning?" Charlie asked.

"Well, there was that girl in El Paso. She was the one that you picked up from Hooter's. Other than her, I don't remember you ever having one in bed in the morning," Abe responded.

"I forgot about that one. She didn't count though. We left her car in the parking lot and I didn't want to have to get dressed and drive her back in the middle of the night. If you remember, you finally drove her and that girl you had back."

"Shit. I forgot about that one. That was the one that made all the noise when we were getting it on, huh?"

"Noise… hell, she was almost screaming," Charlie responded while laughing. "Anyway, Diane is nothing like those other girls. She is special and I will not screw this one up, amigo."

"Okay, boss. I like her too. She doesn't take any shit from anyone. That makes her perfect for you. You never know, it might even help your golf game."

"Speaking of golf," Charlie added. "What do you think about the offer those two guys had from Pecan Valley Country Club?"

"I've never been to Pecan Valley. I think I remember hearing about some guys who went to San Antonio last year. I think they played Pecan Valley but I don't remember what they said about it. Are you still thinking about taking them up on their offer?" Abe asked.

"Yeah," said Charlie. "Now that I'm getting married, I can't expect to be able to support a wife from the little money we make on our little course. They didn't mention anything about money, but it could be pretty good if they give me a percentage of new members, cart fees, lessons and stuff like that. Diane and I will drive up later this week and get more details. If I take the position, I'm serious about bringing you along to make sure we have the best greens in the city. You can have the best golf course in the world, but if the greens are shitty, you're not going to get anyone to play the course. Without new players at the course, you won't have new members sign up."

The two were still talking when Diane walked out of the bathroom with her clothes on and a white towel wrapped around her hair. "The bathroom is all yours," she said.

Abe quickly got up, grabbed his pants lying on the floor and walked gingerly into the bathroom holding his pants in front of his body. "I won't be long," he said as he closed the bathroom door.

Charlie continued to lie in bed watching Diane use the towel to dry her hair as much as possible. She then began putting on her makeup, frequently looking over her shoulder in the mirror at the person watching her from the bed.

"Damn, you're absolutely beautiful," Charlie said quietly.

"Why, thank you," she responded with a teasing smile on her face. "Talk like that will take you far."

"If I say it again, will you get back in bed with me and ravage my body?" he asked.

"Not now. We got a lot of things to do today and there's not enough time. Anyway, Abe will be out of the bathroom in a minute or two."

"How about sending him out for breakfast?" Charlie added.

"If you can get him out of the room for at least thirty minutes, you've got a deal," she said.

That did it with Charlie. He quickly jumped out of bed, put his pants on and pounded on the bathroom door. "Abe, hurry up. I've got to take a piss and you need to go get us breakfast."

"Wait a minute, man. I'll be out in a couple of minutes," Abe shouted through the closed door.

"Hurry up, Abe. You can finish what you have to do later. Right now, you have got to go get breakfast."

Abe opened the door and had a quizzed look on his face. "What's the fucking hurry, man?" he asked.

"Just put your shirt on and go get breakfast. Take your time too," Charlie said while escorting Abe to the door. He grabbed Abe's shirt and shoes, handing them over to Abe. Charlie forced him out of the room before Abe could even put on his shirt. One of the shoes dropped out of Abe's hands and landed on the floor but Charlie quickly kicked it out of the room as he pushed Abe out. "See you in an hour amigo."

Abe was standing at the door, outside the room, holding his shirt and one shoe. He looked down as Charlie kicked the other shoe out of the door. "Dude, this sucks…"

Charlie cut him off, saying, "Abe, just do this for me. I'll see you in an hour."

Before Abe could respond, Charlie closed the door and looked at Diane as she watched through the mirror.

"Abe's gone!" Charlie said with a huge smile on his face. He was now sitting on the edge of the bed.

Diane slowly stepped up and away from the mirror. She turned toward Charlie and said, "This will be one for the record books."

She walked toward Charlie, removing the towel from her hair, and unbuttoned her blouse as she slowly walked to the bed. She stood in front of Charlie, taking her blouse off and tossed it on the other bed.

Charlie started to reach up and grab her but she pushed him back on the bed.

He lay there watching as Diane took off her bra, then her pants. Naked now, she reached down and pulled Charlie's pants off.

15

As she promised, Diane ravaged Charlie's body over and over. With each time, Charlie smiled bigger and bigger like a kid opening up Christmas presents.

Afterwards, the two lay in each other's arms for what seemed like seconds when they were startled by a knock on the door.

"Hey man, it's been an hour. Can I come in?"

It was Abe, who apparently had finished his breakfast.

"Just a minute," Charlie said out loud. He walked to the door as Diane got up and put her clothes back on. She nodded her head when she got back to the mirror and continued to put her makeup on.

Charlie opened the door, allowing Abe to come in.

Abe didn't say anything at first. He brought two Styrofoam cups of coffee and handed them to Charlie. "Here, I brought you guys some coffee."

"Thanks," said Charlie.

"Hey, man. I ran into Hank and some of the other dudes from Lubbock. He's heading back in a few minutes and I'm going to catch a ride with him. You and Diane can then go up to Austin and do whatever you guys need to do. This way, you don't have to explain to Diane's parents why the Mexican is tagging along. It will also give me some time to clear things up at the driving range. If we're not going back there, we need to put some of the equipment up for sale or store it somewhere. Do you want me to see if we can rent the place out to someone?"

"Yeah, I guess. See if Hank or someone else wants to rent the place. If he wants to buy it, get the best price that you can and sell. I'll be out sometime later this week or early next week to get my things. If we need to sign some papers, I can do it then."

16

The plan was now in place. Abe would begin the process of turning the driving range over while Charlie would meet Diane's parents and finalize everything at Pecan Valley.

Charlie and Diane left the Houston area and began the drive to Austin. She called her parents earlier in the day to find out if they would be home as she had some important news to tell them. They said they would be home that afternoon and looked forward to hearing the news.

Diane had told Charlie about her parents and since her father was an avid golfer, she thought the two of them would hit it off quite well. Charlie was nervous but was still looking forward to meeting Diane's parents.

They pulled into the driveway and before they opened the car doors, Diane's parents were coming out of the front door. The smiles on their faces turned to a frown when they noticed their only daughter driving up in an old, rusted out Chrysler.

"Oh, my God," said Diane's mother whispered to her husband.

Using the same, quiet whisper, Diane's father said to his wife, "I'm surprised too, but let's put on the happy face."

"Hi, Mom, Hi Dad," Diane shouted as she opened the car door and stepped out. "It's really great seeing you."

Diane had already walked up to her parents and was giving them both a hug as Charlie walked up from the driveway a bit more slowly. He noticed both of Diane's parents had their eyes focused on him, apparently wondering who he was and why their daughter was bringing him into their lives.

"Mom… Dad, there's someone I want you to meet. This is Charlie Caldwell," Diane said as she reached out and grabbed Charlie's hand. "Charlie, this is my father, Bob Hodor."

Charlie reached out and shook Bob's hand. "It's very good to meet you, Sir. Diane has told me a lot about you."

17

Diane again spoke up and grabbed her mother's hand. "Charlie, this is my Mom. Her name is Lillian but everyone calls her Lil."

Charlie turned toward Diane's mother and offered his hand. "It's really nice to meet you too, Mrs. Hodor. I see where Diane gets her beauty from now."

Diane's mother spoke, "Please Charlie, call me Lil and welcome to our home."

Diane held Charlie's hand as they walked in the front door and into a rather large hallway. Bob and Lil followed them in and motioned them into the main living room.

Diane sat on the sofa and Charlie sat beside her. Both parents took their seats in chairs facing toward the sofa.

Bob broke the short-lived silence. "Charlie, Diane called us from Houston this morning and I guess you guys must be thirsty. Can I bring you a beer or ice tea?"

Charlie wanted to ask for a beer but decided the best approach would be to take the tea. "Sir, I would love a glass of tea."

Diane got up and said, "Mom and I will get it. Dad, are you still drinking Coronas?"

"Yeah, Di, There are some cold ones on the door of the fridge. No lime though," he added.

As the two ladies got up and walked into the kitchen, Charlie nervously looked up and saw Bob's eyes staring at him.

"So, Charlie, tell me a little about yourself. You are the first person Diane has brought to meet us since her high school days. Lil and I both watched you in the Open this weekend. She was so upset. If she could have, she would have reached through the television and grabbed you by the neck. What are your plans now? Are you going to play on the tour?" Bob asked.

18

"Well, Sir… Where do I start? Let's start from a month ago. I had a small driving range near Lubbock and was talked into trying to qualify for the Open this year. I got lucky and found myself playing in Houston. You know how I finished so I want bore you with any of the details on that. I do not have my tour card and really don't think I have the discipline to put in the amount of practice these guys have to do each day."

"So, are you going back to Lubbock?" Bob asked as he continued his questioning.

"Nope, I'm not planning to ever go back to Lubbock. My caddie is out there today and hopefully, he's going to be selling everything we have there. Something very good happened after the tournament on Sunday. The owner of Pecan Valley Country Club in San Antonio offered me the head professional position. That was totally unexpected too. Diane, Abe and I were almost to the car when these two strangers walked up and offered me the job as the head professional. It was totally unexpected."

"That sounds like it could be a great opportunity. Tell me about Pecan Valley. I've played lots of golf in San Antonio but never at a place called Pecan Valley. What kind of membership do they have?" he asked.

"Sir, I really can't tell you much about it. I've never been there but these guys think that I can make some improvements and bring more members in. Diane and I will be driving down there later this week to check it out."

The girls walked back into the room and Bob took the Corona and Charlie had his tea. Lil and Diane were also drinking tea and it was Lil who proposed a toast. "Charlie, welcome to our home."

The group toasted with their glasses and Lil was again the first to speak. "Charlie, I must tell you that I was ready to choke you Sunday. Bob can tell you that I normally do not watch

19

golf but a team of wild horses couldn't have pulled me away from the television that day. Diane told me in the kitchen that she was with you and told you to hit the driver on the tee box. I just have one question... Why the fuck didn't you lay up?"

Charlie looked at Diane for a short time and laughed out loud. He then turned back to Lil. "Lil, I knew I could hit that shot and a million people watching on television didn't think I could pull it off. I told myself that I should lay up, maybe make par and I'd be tied for the lead. My caddie was trying to force an eight-iron into my hands too. I cannot tell you why, but I grabbed the three-wood and hit what I thought was a great shot. I was totally surprised when it fell into the pond. I looked around and my eyes met Diane's." She said "Go for it!""

"Charlie, that's the dumbest thing I've ever heard. Diane doesn't know squat about golf," said Lil with a bit of anger in her voice.

"She certainly knows me and I really needed someone's support. I didn't have it from my fellow players, my caddie or from the crowd. Hell, Abe was ready to kill me," Charlie said. "The only person that really supported me was Diane and nobody knows how much that meant to me."

Diane spoke up. "Mom, I followed Charlie on the last day and I knew the obvious shot was to hit something safe and then try for the birdie or par at worst. Before I met this great man, I would have been in your shoes and taken the safe approach. Now that I know him, I really admire his ability to take a risk and go for it. Once you get to know him, you understand my feelings."

"Maybe," replied Lil. "I still think it was the most stupid thing I've ever witnessed in person or on television."

Diane did not want to continue the conversation concerning the 18th and said, "Okay, let's not talk about the Open. It is history. How are things going for the two of you since dad is completely retired now?"

Lil took the lead and responded, "He plays golf with his group four or five times a week. Basically, it's the same as when he was working only he leaves a bit later in the day."

The conversation continued and everything was pleasant.

The four grilled some steaks for dinner and had a great time sitting around the table. Diane decided this would be the perfect time to give them the news. "Mom… Dad, Charlie has asked me to marry him and I've accepted. We haven't set a date yet but it will be sometime later this year in San Antonio."

Bob and Lil looked at each other with a surprised look on both of their faces.

"Oh," said Lil. "That is something we didn't expect."

Bob turned away from Lil and looked at Charlie. "Are you ready to settle down and take care of my daughter?" he asked.

"Yes, Sir I am. I am more than ready," replied Charlie. "I knew from the very first time I laid eyes on her that she was the one for me. I may not have had the lowest score in the Open, but I can assure you that I was the biggest winner on Sunday when Diane said yes."

Diane and Charlie spent the next two days with Diane's parents and with each day, Bob and Lil Hodor grew more accustomed to having this new person in their lives. They were actually beginning to like him very much. Life was becoming very good for Charlie and Diane.

Chapter Two

Charlie called Pecan Valley and set up Thursday as the day when he would meet with Ned. He wasn't sure what would take place in the meeting but looked forward to seeing the club.

He and Diane made the short drive from Austin and found Pecan Valley without too much problem. They both walked in the pro-shop and walked around looking at merchandise and getting a good first impression of the operation. The young assistant pro behind the counter noticed them when the two entered but didn't say anything.

After several minutes of looking at the various types of golf merchandise, Charlie walked up to the counter.

The assistant stopped what he was doing and said, "Can I help you?"

"Yes," replied Charlie. "What are your green fees for the two of us?"

"We have several types of green fees. If you live in San Antonio, you can get the local rate of $29.00 per round with cart or $17.00 without cart. If you're from out of town, the rates are $35.00 with cart and $24.00 without cart," replied the assistant.

"Why do you increase the rates if someone is from out of town?" Charlie asked.

"I don't know," replied the assistant. "I think the lower rates are to get more locals to play at Pecan Valley."

"Is it working?" asked Charlie.

"I don't know if it works or not. We are getting some people from outside of San Antonio playing the course but most of the time they are with someone from here so they end up paying the reduced rate anyway. If you want, I'll give you the reduced rate even if you're from out of town."

"Okay, give us the reduced rate," said Charlie.

"Are you going to ride?" asked the assistant.

"Yes, we will be riding. We don't have our golf clubs with us. What do you have for rentals?" Charlie asked.

"We have rental clubs available for $15.00 a set. Would you like to get two sets?"

"Yes," said Charlie. "Put us down for two sets. Can you show me what the rentals look like?"

"They're in the back office. Let me get them and I'll be right back," replied the assistant as he left Charlie at the counter and walked in the storage room in the back of the shop.

He soon returned with two old bags with a mix of different types of clubs... different brands and in various states of condition. "Here you go," said the assistant as he handed the two bags over to Charlie.

Charlie looked at the clubs and the bag with a frown on his face. "These clubs are not even the same brand. How can you rent these out to customers?" he asked.

"That's what we have. Do you want to rent them?"

"No, fifteen dollars is too much. Hell, I could go to almost any garage sale and buy a matched set for $15.00. I think we will

24

pass on playing golf. Can you tell me where I can find Mister Wolfolk?" Charlie asked.

"I saw him in the restaurant a few minutes ago. If you go right through the doors on the right, it will take you into the restaurant."

"Okay, thank you," said Charlie. "By the way, what is your name?"

"Brett," replied the assistant.

"Thanks, Brett. We will see you later."

Diane and Charlie walked through the doors and down a short hallway that led to the restaurant. "Well, the pro-shop could use some updating, huh?" Charlie asked.

"The young man behind the counter didn't seem to be very helpful. He needs to work on his customer skills too," Diane added.

The two entered the restaurant and Ned was sitting with a couple of golfers who looked like they just finished playing.

He immediately noticed Charlie and Diane walk in and stood up. "There you are. Did you have any problem finding the golf course?" he asked.

"No, we just followed the map and it brought us right here. I didn't see any signs from the highway though. If we didn't have a map, it would have been a little more difficult," said Charlie.

"That is exactly some of the ideas we're looking for. Charlie, I have some very strong feelings about having you run things for us here at Pecan Valley," said Ned excitingly.

They talked about the trip and discussed the club in general. Later in the conversation, they agreed upon salaries, benefits and other areas that Charlie would be responsible for. They also agreed upon bringing Abe on as the assistant superintendent with what Charlie thought would be an acceptable salary. Charlie would officially become the manager and head professional of the entire facility and would report to Ned directly. He was also going to start on the following Monday.

Following the meeting, Ned took Charlie and Diane around to meet some of the staff working that day. When they went into the pro-shop, Ned introduced Charlie to the assistant behind the counter. "Brett, this is Charlie Caldwell. Charlie will be the new head professional and will be running things at Pecan Valley beginning Monday."

"We met earlier. Welcome on board, Sir," said Brett.

"Glad to be here," replied Charlie. "Officially, I don't start until Monday. In the meantime Brett, think of some things that we can do to make Pecan Valley the place to play golf here in San Antonio."

"I will do, Sir," replied Brett.

"Charlie, I'm not sure if you had the time to find a place to live. In the meantime, we do have a furnished house on the property. It was originally designated to be the superintendents, but it's vacant at the moment. You are more than welcome to stay there as long as you need," said Ned.

Charlie looked at Diane; they were both surprised at the offer. "That sounds good," replied Charlie. "Diane and I will check it out. We were planning on buying a house in the area, but having a free place to stay for the time being would be perfect."

"Okay, let's take a ride," said Ned.

They looked at the house and liked what they saw. It was fairly small but in remarkable condition. It would be perfect for them to live in until they found the right house. They agreed to move in on the next day, Friday.

That evening Charlie looked back on the events of the week with amazement. He went from almost having the lead in the US Open to coming in for fourteenth place. He landed what many professional golfers would call the perfect job. The biggest even by far was finding the girl of his dreams. Charlie Caldwell knew he was truly blessed.

Chapter Three

Charlie walked into the pro-shop early on Monday. Brett was behind the counter and greeted him immediately. "Good morning, Mister Caldwell," he said.

"Good morning," replied Charlie. "And call me Charlie."

"Okay, Charlie. Is there anything that you would like to see first?" Brett asked.

"No, not at the moment, just continue what you do. I'll be walking around and checking things out. I will tell you one thing though… treat everyone that walks through the door as if they're the most important customer you have. Ok? If you can make them feel special, you and I will get along great."

"Yes Sir," replied Brett.

Charlie didn't spend a lot of time in the pro-shop and walked into his small office. It was a mess. Papers, invoices and other items were everywhere. "Where do I start?" Charlie thought to himself.

Not doing anything in the office, Charlie continued his rounds and walked into the restaurant. There were a group of men sitting at one of the tables and one was having breakfast. It was obvious that they were waiting for their tee time so Charlie walked over and introduced himself.

"Hello, guys," said Charlie. "I'm Charlie Caldwell and I'm the new manager of Pecan Valley. You guys must be regulars?"

The group all looked up and one actually stood up and stuck his hand out for a hand shake. "Good to meet you, Charlie. I'm Jim Young," he said.

The others took Jim's lead and all stood up and introduced themselves to Charlie. They all seemed to like it that the new manager actually introduced himself to the group.

Jim continued the conversation. "We were all watching the Open last week and saw the finish. We were actually sitting right over there," pointing to a group of chairs in front of a large TV in the corner. "We were taking bets on if you were going to get one to land on the green."

Charlie smiled and said, "Jim, did you win or lose?"

"I lost five bucks to Hank here. I didn't think you could do it. There had to be so much pressure and then to pull off a shot like that... it was amazing."

"Having to walk through the crowd and across the green, just to turn in a DQ card would have been the real pressure," Charlie replied. "Luckily, that didn't happen."

"I guess," said Jim. "That would have been an impossible walk for me."

"Well, you guys enjoy your round today. Hit them high, far and straight," said Charlie. "By the way, if you guys have any ideas on how we can improve Pecan Valley come and see me. My goal is to make this course the best in the city."

"We will," replied one of the other golfers.

Charlie continued his rounds and walked into the kitchen area. There were two black ladies working and they both looked at him with a surprised look when he walked past the counter and into their space.

"Sir, can I help you?" one asked.

"Yes mam," replied Charlie. "I'm Charlie and the new manager. I would like to try your breakfast this morning. Can you make me two eggs over-easy, bacon, hash-browns and toast?"

"Yes sir," the same one said.

"Thanks. I'm just walking around the kitchen so I can get a good idea of what we have. Is all of the equipment working well?" Charlie asked.

The other lady responded, "The oven leaks so we never really use it. We mostly just cook breakfast and lunch for the golfers. There are other problems too, but we just make do."

"Okay, ladies. Find a piece of paper and as the day goes along, write down any problems you may find and also write down any ideas you have to make things better."

"We will, Sir," replied the first lady. "By the way, my name is Emma and this is Shirley."

Charlie shook both ladies' hands and said, "Glad to meet you both. I really look forward to working with you."

He walked out into the restaurant area and sat down at an empty table. Shirley brought his breakfast out and said, "Here you go, Sir."

"Thank you, Shirley," replied Charlie. "And by the way, call the customers, Sir. Please call me Charlie."

"Okay Charlie. Enjoy your breakfast and let us know if there's anything else we can do."

As other golfers came into the restaurant, they already were told that the new manager was inside. Many took advantage of this information and walked up to Charlie and introduced themselves. Of course, each one wanted to talk about the Open. It was getting old to Charlie, but he didn't mind.

Charlie spent the rest of the day walking around the entire facility and in the afternoon was in the cart barn looking at the golf cart situation.

He didn't notice Abe walk in. "Hey Charlie, the kid in the pro-shop said he thought you'd be in the cart barn. What do you think of this place?"

"Hello Abe," replied Charlie with a huge smile on his face. "Glad you're here. There's a lot of opportunity here and I think we can make it happen. How did everything go in Lubbock?"

"It worked out perfectly. I was trying to rent the place to Hank but he really wasn't interested. Hank and I were talking about temporarily storing the equipment when the Johnson brothers walked in. They flat ass offered one hundred thousand dollars for everything."

Charlie stopped him, "One hundred thousand! Wow, that was going to be my asking price. So, what did you say?"

"You would have been proud of me, Charlie," Abe said. "I acted like I was choking and said, one hundred thousand? That would be Ok for the land but what about the equipment. You know, we got fairway mowers, greens mowers and a tractor. Plus we have fifteen golf carts. That equipment is worth fifty thousand. Bottom line is that I sold everything for

31

one hundred and thirty thousand dollars to the Johnson brothers."

"The Johnson brothers?" questioned Charlie. "They don't know a fucking thing about golf or golf courses."

"I know that. The dudes say that they have a cousin who just got his PGA Apprentice card and he will be running the place. I didn't meet the cousin but we don't have to worry because it now belongs to them," replied Abe.

"How did they pay?" Charlie asked.

"That's the best part Charlie. They gave me a cashier's check and it cleared the bank. The money is in our account we used for the course."

"That is absolutely fantastic," replied Charlie. "You did a great job with that, Abe."

"How are things at this course?" Abe asked.

"Not too bad," Charlie replied. "I've checked out most of the carts. They're not in too bad shape either. A couple of them need new batteries but most seem to be running well. I also made a quick check of the mowing equipment. It's all in good shape too. I'll let you take a closer look though. The superintendent they have seems to be a pretty good guy. I looked at one of the greens and it wasn't too bad either. Again, I'll rely on you to give it a more thorough check. I was just about ready to jump in a cart and take a drive around the course. Want to go?"

"Let's do it," said Abe.

The two drove around the course and met golfers in several other groups. Each time Charlie introduced himself and they all wanted to talk about the Open. Charlie gave them all the same answer.

Abe concentrated on the condition of the course. He was looking at everything, including greens, bunkers, tee boxes and fairways. Everything seemed to be in fairly good condition. The bunkers could use some work but overall, he was very happy with what he looked at.

As the two were riding back to the cart barn, Charlie asked, "Well, what is your opinion of the course condition?"

"It's not bad," replied Abe. "The superintendent is doing a pretty good job. We can certainly do a few things here and there, but overall, the course is in good shape."

Charlie introduced Abe to Chuck Hardy, the superintendent. "Chuck, this is Abe. He worked with me in Lubbock and we had the best greens in West Texas. He says you've done a great job here so with the two of you, I expect Pecan Valley to have the best greens in Texas next year."

Abe stayed with Chuck and they went over the equipment with a fine-toothed comb. Meanwhile, Charlie went back to the pro-shop and met the other assistant. Dave Lopez was behind the counter with Brett when Charlie walked in.

Dave took the initiative and said, "Hello Charlie. Brett told me a little about you and I'm glad to see new management. Is there anything I can do for you at the moment?"

"Good to meet you, Dave," said Charlie. "Since business seems to be a bit slow at the moment, let's discuss some ideas I see as an immediate improvement."

"First of all, let's talk about our price structure. When I came in last week, Brett thought that I was just another out of town

33

customer. He told me about the pricing and I was lost. We need to have a simple price structure but make it a deal for golfers to join. Let's come up with a plan where it's a no-brainer for them to join the club as members. You two know more about the current pricing here in San Antonio so put your heads together and be ready to give me some ideas on pricing by Wednesday. I want to increase our number of members by three hundred by the end of the year."

Brett looked at Charlie, then at Dave. "Three hundred new members is a huge increase. I don't know if that will be possible," he said.

"Nothing is impossible," replied Charlie. "Thousands of people thought that hitting your last ball two-hundred and forty-seven yards to an island green was impossible. Nothing is impossible and I expect you to make it happen."

"Okay Charlie, we'll come up with something," replied Dave.

"Now, let's talk about you two and your salary. I know that assistants don't make squat. I can't really do much about the salary but think I can generate some additional income with passing lessons off to each of you. When you have lessons, I will step in and work the counter."

"What percentage do we get from lessons?" Brett asked.

"What was the percentage before?"

"We were allowed to keep seventy-five percent. Twenty-five went back to the club to cover our time from being away from the counter," Brett added.

"Well, since I will be covering you on the counter, you should be able to keep it all, huh? The only thing I ask is that you make every attempt to schedule any lessons during periods when we're slow or when you're off. I understand that this may not be the case all the time so I'll be there to cover."

"Thank you, Charlie," said Brett. "That will be very helpful."

"Yeah, thanks," Dave added.

The first day at the club was over and Charlie was happy with everything they accomplished. He met many golfers and was pleased with the staff at the club. Ned was providing a budget to make some necessary changes and Charlie felt very good.

When Charlie got back to the house, Diane was beaming. She went house-hunting and found a beautiful home just a few miles from the course. With the money due to come in from the Open, they should have enough for a down payment. Charlie went with Diane and they looked at the house together. It was a fairly new house, had a great floor-plan and was fairly close to the course.

"I like it," said Charlie. "You did real well in finding it and picking it out. We won't have to wait until the Open check comes either. Abe came back from Lubbock this afternoon and he sold the course there for one hundred and thirty thousand dollars. Abe and I owned it together so we have sixty-five thousand to play with. I say let's go for it."

Chapter Four

Within several months, Charlie was making huge strides with the club. It was rated as one of the top 100 courses in the State and this was great news. Memberships increased but not to the level expected. Charlie spoke with one of the members who was affiliated with one of the local television stations. The station agreed to do an interview on the new Pecan Valley and the new Head Professional.

The interview was more focused on the Open but Charlie was happy with that… as long as the end result was more members. It was a huge hit as golfers from all around wanted the chance to meet Charlie. Of course Charlie would convince many of them that they were able to get the golfing deal of a lifetime at Pecan Valley and within a few weeks, the membership grew by over four hundred.

Abe and Chuck worked well together. Though Abe was the assistant superintendent, he and Chuck treated each other as equals. The course conditions continued to improve and soon Pecan Valley greens were generally thought of as the best in San Antonio for sure and some of the best in the State.

Additional folks were hired for the restaurant and it was all placed under the supervision of Shirley. She listened to customers and made every attempt to provide them with quality food when they demanded it. Members were actually eating there and the food was absolutely great. Under Shirley's direction, the restaurant was generating more profit than ever before.

The pro-shop had the biggest improvement. Merchandise was priced affordable and most of it quickly moved off the shelves. Two additional employees were added and they covered Brett and Dave when lessons were being conducted.

Ned offered Charlie a substantial raise as a bonus and Charlie requested that the extra money be passed on to the workers as raises. Ned agreed to this but also gave Charlie the raise offered.

Everything was great in Charlie and Diane's lives. They had a new house, new furniture and even a new car that was given by Diane's parents as an early wedding present.

The only surprising news was Diane's announcement that she was pregnant. Though both she and Charlie thought this was great news, it required a change in their plans to get married. Instead of waiting until the summer of next year, the date moved up to thirty days.

Diane's mother came down and helped with the wedding plans. It was going to be held at the club and looked like it was going to be the biggest event ever. Over three hundred guests showed up and the ceremony was conducted on the 18th green. It was an absolutely beautiful ceremony.

Charlie continued to grow and improve Pecan Valley. Membership levels were fairly consistent and the club continued to make considerable amounts of money each year.

Charlie and Diane's life at home also improved considerably. Michael Robert Caldwell was born on the 21st of June. The birth went perfectly and mother and son were soon at home with the happy father.

Through the next several years, there were some improvements made to the club. The club was changed from a private club to a semi-private club. This was a minor change as Pecan Valley always accepted play from non-members.

Abe became the head superintendent when Chuck Hardy moved to a different club. However, that move did not have any effect on the quality of the greens at Pecan Valley. They were still considered to be some of the best greens in Texas.

Pecan Valley continued its steady growth as did its reputation as one of the premier places to play golf in San Antonio. Membership met and maintained its goal of being over ninety-five percent full. Bonuses were frequently passed out to employees across the board and the club was also known as the place to work in South Texas if you were in the golf profession.

Robert Michael grew up at the golf course. He went by his middle name and everyone just called him Mikey. Mikey played golf quite well but did not have the fire in his belly to approach a career in professional golf. That was just fine with his mother and father. Deep inside, Charlie hoped Mikey would have the same love for the game as he did, but that wasn't to be.

Mikey graduated from high school and decided he wanted to be a teacher. He was attending the University of Texas in Austin hoping to earn a position teaching physical education at one of the high schools in Austin.

Life was good for Charlie and Diane as they entered their senior years.

Chapter Five

As he grew older, Charlie began having memory problems. He couldn't remember names very well but thought that this was natural with everyone. He would also forget birthdays and his anniversary. Again, he didn't put much thought or concern in this as he thought it was just natural.

Charlie's first indication of serious memory problems was at an awards presentation for the Pecan Valley Club Championship. As usual, the last award was to the golfer who won the championship. Charlie grabbed the trophy and announced, "This year's winner with a score of two twenty-one for three days is…" He paused on the name as he was looking at the golfer right in front of him. For the life of him, Charlie could not figure out what his name was!

Totally flustered and embarrassed, Charlie looked quickly around the room before saying loudly, "Mister Two Twenty-One!"

The crowd clapped and most didn't even catch the slip-up. Charlie caught it though and afterwards, sitting at the table, tried harder and harder to come up with the winning golfer's name. He'd known this golfer for several years and had seen him in the club many times this past week. Each time, Charlie acknowledged him by name. However, tonight, the golfer's name was a complete blank.

After the awards ceremony, Charlie went into his office to put things away before closing the shop and heading home. He was still trying to remember the name and it seemed the harder he tried to think of the name, the further away he was from remembering it. "God-damn, why can't I remember his name?" Charlie quietly asked himself.

He related the story to Diane when he got home. At first, he hesitated telling her because Diane frequently took things to the extreme. "Hon, I have to tell you this. I had a very embarrassing moment this evening," he said.

"What happened?" Diane asked.

"Well, Bobby Holiday won the Club Championship and when I was giving him his trophy, I could not remember his name. Bobby Holiday! I've known this kid for years but for some reason I couldn't think of it tonight. I stumbled during the announcement and looked at the audience while I frantically tried to think of his name. God, it was embarrassing, too. Finally, I just called him Mister Two Twenty-One since that was his score."

"Did they buy it?" she asked.

"Yeah, I think so," said Charlie. Continuing, he added, "Even afterwards in the office, and in the car on the way home, I tried to remember his name. It was impossible and only when I started telling you about what happened, the name of Bobby Holiday popped out."

"You sound worried about this, hon. It's probably just from the stress of running another great tournament," Diane added.

"God, I hope so," replied Charlie. "You know, I seem to be getting worse and worse with names these days. Someone introduces themselves to me and as they are walking away, I can't even remember their names. I'm worried."

"It happens to all of us," Diane said.

A few days later, Charlie was making his routine drive around the course, checking things out. He noticed that certain areas were changing color from the bright green to a dull brown. "Damn, I reminded Abe last week to begin fertilizing," he thought to himself.

Charlie stopped by the maintenance shed and caught Abe working on one of the mowers. "Abe, how's it going?" he asked.

"Oh, hey Charlie," Abe said looking up from the mower. "One of the blades on this mower caught a bolt and I'm just replacing it," he added.

"Abe, I told you last week to start fertilizing. Why didn't you get on it? Things are starting to turn brown on us."

Abe looked at Charlie with a surprised face. "Charlie, we talked about this yesterday. Don't you remember, we agreed to start in on Monday?" Abe responded.

"I didn't talk to you about this, Abe," said Charlie with a bit of anger in his voice.

"You certainly did. We were driving around the course and we talked about it for a good thirty minutes. Don't you remember? We're going to try the new fertilizer from Ortho?"

The term "Ortho" must have jogged Charlie's memory as it came back to him. Slowly, he began to remember the events that took place between he and Abe. "Oh yeah, I remember now," said Charlie.

"Still want to start it Monday?" Abe asked.

"Yeah, Monday will be fine," Charlie answered.

41

Charlie got back in the cart and drove slowly back to the pro-shop but couldn't believe that he completely forgot about the conversation about fertilizing.

At first Abe didn't think anything about Charlie's memory lapse but it continued to bother him. He decided to check it out further and drove a golf cart up to Charlie's office.

When he walked into Charlie's office, Abe looked at him for a moment.

"What's up, Abe?" Charlie asked.

"Nothing much," replied Charlie. "I am a little worried about you though."

"Oh, the fertilizer thing, don't let that worry you," said Charlie. "I've been a bit forgetful lately and it must be that I'm not getting enough sleep. Hell, I even forgot Bobby's name during the award presentation for this year's club championship."

"How could you have forgotten Bobby's name? Hell, he's around here almost every day."

"I don't know," said Charlie. "I just had a complete blank and couldn't think of his name no matter how hard I tried."

"Charlie, you might want to see someone about this," said Abe with a concerned tone in his voice.

"Nah, it will be Ok. I'll get a good night's sleep tonight and it will be better tomorrow. I guarantee it," said Charlie.

"Okay, sorry to bring it up but I was just concerned."

Abe left and Charlie was a bit concerned. He knew that he was having harder and harder times trying to remember things, but simply attributed it to stress and lack of sleep.

Things seemed to be better for Charlie the next few days and any memory problem Charlie seemed to have been corrected by getting more sleep.

Charlie was still asleep on Sunday when the phone rang at 7:30am. It was Shirley from the restaurant. "Mister Caldwell, this is Shirley. We have dozens of golfers here and the pro-shop isn't open. They asked me about it but I cannot open the pro-shop. That's why I'm calling you."

"The pro-shop isn't open?" he questioned Shirley.

"No Sir. Normally, Brett has it open by 6am but not today. It's locked up tighter than a drum. The starters have put some golfers out but I thought you should know," Shirley said.

"Okay, I got it and will be there in a few minutes," said Charlie.

As he was driving to the course, Charlie was worried about Brett. He was also angry with Brett for not opening up or at the very least, calling in.

Charlie arrived at the club and walked quickly to the pro-shop where several golfers were waiting. One of them made a joking comment by saying "Good afternoon, Charlie."

This really pissed-off Charlie and he cursed Brett under his breath. "I'll have everything ready to go in a minute or so," he answered. "Brett was supposed to be here but something must have come up."

Charlie opened the shop and got the golfers checked in. As soon as he had a free moment, he called Brett's home phone number. Brett's girlfriend answered the phone and said, "Hello."

"This is Charlie at the course. Is Brett Ok?" he asked.

"I don't know. Is something wrong?" she asked.

"Well, he didn't show up for work today and I thought he must have slept in."

"No, he didn't sleep in. He and his brother went down to Padre Island last night. They were supposed to be going fishing today," she said. "Is Brett Ok?"

"I didn't know he was going fishing," Charlie said. "He's scheduled to work today."

"Brett said that he had the day off and has been planning this for several weeks. Are you sure he was supposed to be at work today?"

"His name is on the schedule," Charlie said as he held the schedule in front of him. He then looked at today's date and sure enough, it showed Brett to be gone and Charlie was supposed to open. "I take that back. I see that Charlie had changed the schedule and put me down to open up. When Brett returns have him give me a call."

"Okay, I will have Brett call you Mister Caldwell," replied Brett's girlfriend.

Charlie thought about Brett and having the day off but couldn't remember him talking about it. He was convinced that Brett never mentioned this to him and was upset that Brett took the day off without ever having talked to him.

44

The next day, Charlie received a call from Brett, who was still at Padre Island. "Charlie, I just spoke with Nadine and she told me that you wanted me to call you. Is everything Ok?"

"Not really," said Charlie. "You changed the schedule without telling me about it. You were supposed to open yesterday."

"Charlie, we talked about this last week. I told you that my brother was coming into town and we were going to fishing in the Gulf. You told me that there wouldn't be any problem and you would cover for me on Sunday. Don't you remember?" Brett asked.

"No, I don't remember that conversation and would have certainly remembered since Sunday is one of our busiest days around here. We'll talk about it when you come back," said Charlie.

"Do you need me to drive back up today?" Brett asked.

"No, go ahead and catch some fish. I see on the schedule that you will be in on Wednesday. We'll talk then."

"Okay, see you on Wednesday," Brett said as he hung up the phone.

Charlie tried to remember the conversation that he and Brett had but couldn't remember anything about him taking the day off and going fishing. Charlie was convinced that Brett simply took the day off and changed the schedule without telling him.

On Wednesday, Charlie confronted Brett. "Brett, I thought about it for the last few days and do not remember you mentioning anything about going fishing. I'm going to give you the day off Sunday but do not ever let this happen again. Understand?"

"Sir, we did talk about it. I would never miss a day on purpose and leave you hanging, especially on a Sunday," Brett said.

"Brett, we did not talk about it. I would have remembered that conversation. So let's drop it."

"Okay Sir, I'll drop it. However, you might check with Abe as he was with you when I asked you about taking the day off."

Charlie thought that Abe could straighten things out and drove a cart down to the cart barn where Abe was working on one of the golf carts.

"Abe, do you remember a conversation between Brett and me concerning him going fishing Sunday?" Charlie asked.

"Yeah, is he back?" questioned Abe. "He was going to bring back some Red Fish."

"Yeah, he's back," said Charlie.

"I must have forgotten about the conversation. I was ready to fire him for not showing up for work on Sunday. Thanks, I'll go back up and apologize to him for raking him over the coals."

Charlie walked back into the pro-shop and was a bit embarrassed as he saw Brett. "Brett, please accept my apologies. I just talked with Abe and he remembered the conversation concerning your brother coming to San Antonio and the two of you going fishing. I've been a bit forgetful lately and our conversation just slipped my mind."

"No problem, Mister Caldwell," replied Brett.

As the days progressed, Charlie's memory problems became more and more common. He forgot simple things like how to make a price correction in the cash register and had to get Brett to complete the transaction. He was also constantly forgetting where he set something down.

Most of the staff noticed this, but because of Charlie's status at the club, these lapses in memory were not brought up.

Diane also noticed Charlie's deteriorating memory too. Charlie would frequently forget simple things around the house. He constantly forgot where he put things and was always asking Diane to help find these items.

Diane was concerned and decided to bring it up to Charlie one day. "Hon, you seem to be forgetting more and more things lately. How about making an appointment to have your memory checked out?" she asked.

"I don't have a memory problem," replied Charlie in an angry voice. "I'm getting sick and tired of people telling me that I have a memory problem. Hell, I'm just getting old and everyone has memory issues as they get up in years. Mine is no different."

"Don't get angry with me, hon. I'm just worried about you and it wouldn't take very long to have everything checked. Can I make an appointment for you?" Diane asked.

"Hell no," shouted Charlie. "I don't need to pay someone to tell me that I'm getting old and also getting forgetful. I won't go to a doctor."

Deciding that it would be useless to continue the conversation, Diane decided to drop the matter for the moment.

After Charlie left for work the next day, Diane called Mikey and told him about Charlie's lapse in memory.

"Mom, I don't think you have to worry about Dad. He's just getting a bit more forgetful as he gets older. It happens to most people. Hell, I'm even forgetful at times," Mikey said.

The conversation with Mikey reassured her that there probably wasn't any problem at all. Though she was still aware of memory issues, she didn't think nothing serious was wrong.

A more serious issue occurred a few days later. Charlie was working for one of the assistants and was going to close the shop. Abe was also working late in the cart barn and when he drove past the pro-shop around eight pm, he saw the lights were still on. He stopped and thought he'd share a beer with Charlie since he was also working late. Abe walked into the pro-shop and it was empty. The registers were still open but no one was there. Abe walked outside and the parking lot was empty.

Thinking something bad had happened, Abe called Charlie's house. Charlie answered, "Hello."

"Hey Charlie, any reason no one closed up the pro-shop today?" Abe asked.

"I closed the pro-shop, Abe," said Charlie.

"Well, guess where I'm calling you from?" Abe asked sarcastically. "I'm standing in front of one of the registers and it's open."

"You're shitting me. Abe, I was certain I closed everything... or at least I thought I did. I'll be right down and close up. Wait for me there, Ok?"

"I'll be here," said Abe.

Charlie was there in a few minutes and had a strange look on his face when he walked in. He was obviously very nervous. Later, he tried to run the end of day routine on the registers to get the day's results. Charlie was flustered and it showed. He was almost on the verge of panicking as he made mistake after mistake. Finally, he had everything completed and put the cash in the safe.

Abe was watching everything and was really worried for his friend. He was pained by watching Charlie making common mistakes and when Abe offered to help, he was shunned. After everything was complete, Abe finally confronted Charlie.

"Man, something is going on with you, Charlie. You need to see someone," Abe said. "They have drugs that can help with your memory issues."

"Abe, I just forgot to close. I was doing something and simply thought I had already closed the pro-shop. I got in my car and drove home. This isn't that big of a deal," he added.

"It would have been a big deal if I hadn't found the pro-shop open. What if Joe Blow from the street walked up to find an opened pro-shop? He'd have all the cash and at least ten sets of new golf clubs, plus enough shirts to wear for a year of two. Charlie, it is a big deal and you have got to do something about it."

"Fuck you, Abe. You wouldn't have this job if I wouldn't have stood up for you. Now that I need you to stand up for me, you want to throw me under the bus," replied Charlie.

"Hey man, don't get nasty on me. I'm your friend and just trying to watch out for you," said Abe.

"Well, it's over and done with. The shop's closed now so I'm going home. You can do whatever you want."

Abe watched his friend get in his car and drive home. He was really concerned with Charlie now.

Diane tried to find out from Charlie why he had to go back to the club but Charlie refused to tell her the real reason. Later that night, she called Abe and he told her what had happened.

The next day, she contacted Ned Wolfolk and mentioned that she was concerned with her husband and did not want him to be in a position where his memory or lack of memory caused the club any major problems.

Ned understood and said he would check into it. Ned had not been to Pecan Valley in some time but thought it would be good to stop by and see Charlie.

The next day, Ned drove down from Austin and walked into the pro-shop. Brett recognized Ned and greeted him as he walked in. "Good morning, Mister Wolfolk."

"Good morning, Brett. Is Charlie in?" he asked.

"Yes, I believe he's in his office," Brett said pointing to Charlie's office.

"Thanks, I'll just walk in on him."

Ned walked into Charlie's office and Charlie looked up. Charlie recognized him but couldn't remember his name. "Hey, good morning, what brings you out our way?" Charlie asked.

"I was just making my rounds and it has been some time since I've been back to Pecan Valley. We have several more clubs now and they seem to be giving us problems. We haven't had any problems here so we've just left everything up to you.

You and your staff are doing a great job for us. Let's walk around," Ned suggested.

"Sure, I'll show you some of the things we've got going on here," replied Charlie.

The two walked through the restaurant and out to the putting green where several golfers were putting while they waited for their tee time. One of the golfers was Bobby Holiday and he recognized Charlie and walked up.

Charlie saw him walk up and said, "Hey Bobby, getting ready for another sub-par round?"

"We will see. I just wanted to tell you thanks for running a great club championship tournament. It was great," Bobby said, looking at the person standing next to Charlie. "Hi, I'm Bobby Holiday."

Charlie couldn't avoid it. "Excuse me, Bobby this is one of the owners of Pecan Valley," he said pausing for an agonizing three or four seconds. "Your first name is one the tip of my tongue," again pausing.

Ned broke Charlie's silence and said, "Hi Bobby, I'm Ned Wolfolk. I've come up for the day to see how things are going. It's nice to meet you. Now, go take their money."

"We'll try for sure," Bobby said as he walked back to the putting green.

There was a long bit of silence between Charlie and Ned. Charlie broke the ice and said, "Ned, I'm sorry about temporarily forgetting your name. I've been having some problems with my memory lately and it has a lot of people concerned. Diane thinks I should get it checked out but I think it's only part of getting old."

51

"Diane may be right. If it is something, the sooner they discover it the better they can treat it. Charlie, we have an excellent doctor in Austin that specializes in memory issues. Why don't you come up to see him for an evaluation?" Ned suggested.

"It will probably be a waste of time but I'll do it," Charlie said.

A few minutes later, the two were back in Charlie's office and Ned called his office and had his secretary make an appointment for Charlie to see the doctor. Within minutes she had an appointment set up for next Monday.

Chapter Six

Charlie and Diane drove to Austin the meet with Dr. Freeman, who specializes in dementia problems.

They were called into the office and Dr. Freeman introduced himself and asked Charlie why he thought he was at the doctor's office.

"People think that I have memory problems but I don't think my memory issues are anything more than any other person over fifty-five has. I forget things, but who doesn't?" he asked.

"You're right, Charlie," the doctor responded. "As we all get older, we tend to forget things. However, occasionally we may forget more things that are normally remembered. I've looked at your family history and there's no mention of severe dementia. That's good and bad. If there was a history, we'd have something to go on. In your case, there's no history so we have to start from scratch."

"As far as I know, my parents or their parents did not have dementia. My Mom had an excellent memory until the day she died at seventy-two," Charlie added.

"That's good to know, Charlie," responded the doctor. "Tell me some of the things that have happened recently that may have caused you concern."

"Well, I forget names all the time. But, who doesn't? I also forget some things that people have told me. That is a problem at home and at work. I also forgot to close our pro-shop one day and that could have been a big problem."

"I see," said the doctor. "Well, Charlie, I'm going to run a few tests on you. These tests are simple problems that are designed to test your temporary memory… you know, the type of things that everyone should be able to do easily. Are you ready to begin?"

"Yeah, I guess," said Charlie.

Diane remained in the waiting area while Charlie and the doctor went into another office.

After both Charlie and doctor sat down, the doctor asked if he was ready to begin.

"Yeah, let's get it over with," said Charlie.

"Okay, the first problem is simple, Charlie. I want you to count backwards from one hundred in increments of seven. For example, you would say one hundred then ninety-three, eighty-six and so on. When you're ready, you can start."

"Hell, this is easy," Charlie said. "One-hundred, ninety-three, eighty-six, eighty-nine… no, not eighty-nine, let's start over. I can do this, I know. Ok… one-hundred, ninety-three, eight-six, seventy-nine, seventy-two, seventy-nine… Damn, this is harder than I thought."

"Okay, Charlie that was more of a coordination test. I'm going to read five words to you and I want you to remember them. Are you ready?" the doctor asked.

"Go ahead," said Charlie.

"Okay, Elephant, snowman, airplane, statue and television," the doctor said, pausing a few seconds between each word. "Now Charlie, tell me the third word."

Charlie didn't expect to have to tell the words back this way and was completely lost. He could remember elephant. What followed elephant? he asked himself. "Let's see," he said out loud. Elephant was the first word, and then there was airplane... wait a minute, something else was before this. After a few minutes, Charlie gave up, saying, "This is a stupid test."

"You sound like you're a bit frustrated, Charlie. Would you like to take a few moments before we conduct the next test?" the doctor asked.

"No, let's get it over with," said Charlie in a frustrated tone.

"Okay, Charlie, I want you to draw a clock and show the time to be as near as possible to three thirty-five. Just draw the face of the clock as a circle and do not put numbers on it. Here's a pencil and paper. Do you understand the instructions?"

"Yes, I understand. That's easy," said Charlie. He drew a circle and in the center drew the hour hand pointing to the three. He drew the minute hand and it pointed to the bottom of the face. However, the hour hand was much longer than the minute hand. "There, the time is three-thirty four."

The doctor looked at the clock Charlie drew but didn't say anything. "Great Charlie, now we'll take the last test for today." The doctor reached into his pocket and took out some change. There were three quarters, two dimes, four nickels and six pennies. "Charlie, I would like for you to study these coins."

Charlie counted the coins and came up with one dollar and twenty-one cents. "Okay, I got it," said Charlie.

The doctor put a piece of paper over the coins and asked, "Whose portrait is on the quarter?"

This question caught Charlie by surprise. He thought about it and after a few seconds, he knew whose portrait was on the quarter. "George Washington," he said.

"That's correct and now tell me how much money is there adding up all the coins?" asked the doctor.

Charlie knew he had the answer just a second ago but couldn't remember what it was. He was again getting frustrated. "Let's see, there were three quarters, which is seventy-five cents. Was there two nickels and two dimes?" he asked himself out loud. Finally, after a few moments, he threw out a guess. "One dollar and six cents," he answered.

The doctor pulled back the paper, revealing the coins.

Charlie realized he miscounted the nickels and dimes. "Shit, I knew that," he said.

The doctor terminated the test and they went back to the office where he called Diane into the room.

"Charlie, the test we went through today was designed to test a person's short-term memory. The results show that you have some issues concerning short-term memory. However, I cannot confirm dementia at this time nor can I tell you what is causing your memory loss. I am going to refer you to a good neurologist. He's one of the best in the country and he will conduct a full physical to see if there is a medical condition that could be causing your memory issues. I'll have my secretary make an appointment so you can get this completed as soon as possible. As with anything, the earlier you can get a diagnosis, the better the results will be for treating it. Are you good with this?" he asked.

"Yes, I can tell you that I should have been able to pass your tests today so I know something is wrong. Let's find out what it is and get it fixed," Charlie said.

Charlie was able to get an appointment with the neurologist the next morning.

The neurologist did a complete blood work, physical exam and lastly did a CT scan on Charlie's upper body. The results were quickly made available and the neurologist discussed the results with both, Charlie and Diane.

"Mister Caldwell," the neurologist said. "The CT scan we conducted this morning is only one of the tools we can use to diagnose changes in the brain. One of the things we look for is any signs that the brain may be shrinking. You scan shows a slight space between the skull and Dura matter surrounding the brain. This may be as a result of the onset of Alzheimer's. However, there are certainly other reasons for slight shrinkage in the brain so this is not a confirmation that you, in fact, have Alzheimer's."

"Alzheimer's," Charlie questioned the doctor. "I can't have Alzheimer's. Hell, I'm only fifty-five."

"Sir, most patients do not develop Alzheimer's until their middle sixties but it's not uncommon for the disease to show up in some patients as early as forty or forty-one."

Diane spoke up with a question, "I read some articles on Alzheimer's and they say there's no cure at the moment but progress is being made with certain drugs that can slow the disease's progress. Is that true?"

The neurologist looked at Diane and then at Charlie, "There are many groups and medical facilities that are studying Alzheimer's. Some drugs seem to slow the progress in some patients but these drugs do not seem to have an effect on others. We simply do not know enough about it at this time."

"How can we tell if I have it for sure?" Charlie asked.

"Sir, there's no test that will confirm diagnosis for sure," the doctor replied.

"Let's say that I do have the beginning stages of Alzheimer's. What would be my time?" Charlie asked intently.

"Well, there's nothing standard about Alzheimer's. It affects people differently. In some cases, patients lose coordination very quickly, while others seem to retain coordination and the ability to function with limitations. I have one patient that has had Alzheimer's for several years. She has problems recognizing her family members, but she can sit down at a piano and play classical music from memory. I have another that loves to bowl. This man can throw strike after strike but has no idea how to keep his score. As you can see, there's nothing I can tell you that can confirm you have it for sure or what will be the outcome. The best advice I can give you is to stay as active as possible."

Charlie looked a bit more positive and said, "Thank you doctor."

They left the neurologist's office and headed home to San Antonio, stopping by a drug store to get the neurologist's prescription filled. When they arrived home, Charlie walked in the back yard and sat down in one of the lounge chairs.

Diane fixed two glasses of tea and joined her husband.

Charlie was softly crying, tears streaming down his face. This started some tears from Diane.

She set the tea down and reached over and hugged her love. "Hon, it will be Ok. We'll get through this one day at a time."

Charlie looked up at his loving wife and didn't say anything. He only slightly nodded his head.

They discussed what they wanted to do to get through this and both decided that Charlie should quit working at the golf course. He loved going in but his memory problems would eventually become a problem for himself and for the club. They decided it would best for him to just not go in as the manager.

Diane passed this decision to Ned in a phone call and he told her that this was probably the best decision that could be made. "Diane, this would be best for Charlie and for the club. Everyone at the club and in the organization loves Charlie and will provide any support we can. Of course, if Charlie's condition would improve, he would always be welcome at the club," said Ned.

Diane thanked him, and hung up the phone.

During the next few weeks, Charlie would frequently go to the club, have lunch and spend an hour or so hitting golf balls on the range. He didn't have the distance he once had but was able to make fairly solid contact. It felt good when he hit one in the center of the club face and allowed him to forget his condition.

After one outing at the club, Charlie was in his car heading home. "Something was wrong," he thought. "This doesn't look right." He didn't recognize the street or the buildings. He missed his turn. He drove around for a couple of hours trying to find his home but he kept getting farther and farther away. Soon, he was on the opposite side of San Antonio and was almost out of gas. Not knowing what to do, he decided to stop the car and figure out where he was at. Unfortunately, he stopped in the middle of one of the busy freeways in the city. Cars were swerving by on the left and right but one didn't quite make it around and clipped the side of Charlie's car. This cause Charlie's car to spin and it was again hit by another car. Soon, several cars were involved and traffic came to a complete halt.

Charlie stayed in his car holding the steering wheel tight. He was nervous and afraid. Fortunately, no one was injured in the accident and one of the drivers walked up to Charlie's car and knocked on the window. Charlie, rolled down the window and said, "I'm sorry, I got lost. I'm sorry… I'm sorry."

Soon, a policeman arrived on the scene and asked Charlie to get out of the car, which he did. The policeman obviously thought alcohol was involved but quickly realized that Charlie had not been drinking. An ambulance arrived on the scene and soon Charlie found himself on the way to the hospital.

Diane was called and quickly made her way to the hospital where she found Charlie sitting in a chair in the waiting room. He saw her when she walked in and stood up to meet her.

"What happened, Charlie?" she asked.

"I don't know," replied Charlie. "I must have missed a turn. I kept driving trying to find some building or street so I could figure out where I was. Nothing looked familiar. They say I stopped in the middle of the freeway when I was suddenly hit by a car and then hit by another car. Next thing I know was that I was brought here to the hospital. The doctor looked me over and said there was nothing wrong and released me. I'm sorry," he added as he began to cry.

Diane hugged him and tried to reassure him. "Charlie, this could have happened to anyone. Let's go home," she suggested.

Diane helped Charlie to his feet and she held his hand tightly as they walked to the car. When they arrived home, there were several messages from the police and insurance company. Everyone wanted to know what exactly happened.

Diane took care of everything, but didn't have Charlie's car replaced. She obviously realized that this was a sign that Charlie shouldn't be driving alone any longer.

Charlie still wanted to go to the golf course frequently so Diane drove him there and would pick him up a few hours later. Occasionally, Abe would bring him home. However, Charlie would not be driving there again.

Other problems seemed to creep up on Charlie. He would forget simple things like brushing his teeth, shaving and other things he should be doing each day. Diane was becoming a full-time caregiver and it was taking a toll on her. Her life was being consumed by Charlie and she realized that eventually it would change her for the worse. That was when she realized she needed help. Mikey was the only choice she had and she called him with a plea to help.

Chapter Seven

Diane called Mikey that evening. When he answered, the two talked about school and eventually it came around to talking about Charlie. "Mikey, I don't think I can manage your father much longer. I'm getting older too and there is just too much pressure on me to make sure he brushes his teeth, cleans himself when he goes to the bathroom, watch to be sure he doesn't walk off somewhere. It's a 24 hour a day job and I need your help."

Mikey didn't have to think on this. "Mom, I can certainly help. I'll drive down this weekend and we'll talk things out, Ok?" he asked rhetorically.

"Can you come down any sooner?" Diane asked. "I need some help immediately. I'm really afraid that I'm going to do something that I'll regret or that Charlie is going to do something to hurt himself."

"Sure, I can be down in a couple of hours. Let me tidy things up around my apartment and I'll leave in an hour or so," he said. "Mom, just relax for an hour or so and I'll be right down."

Mikey showed up as promised and as he walked into the house, he saw his dad watching television. His dad looked up and Mikey wasn't sure he recognized who he was. "Hi Dad, how are you tonight?" he asked.

Charlie was still looking at the young man and suddenly recognized who just walked in. "Hello Mikey, what a surprise.

Does your Mom know you're here?" Charlie asked. "Diane… Diane, Mikey is here."

Diane came from the back bedroom and hugged Mikey quite hard and long. "God, I'm glad you're here," she said.

"I'm glad too," replied Mikey.

Charlie went back to watching his television show and was oblivious to his wife and son talking in the kitchen.

"Mikey, I cannot keep up with him. He's constantly getting into things and gets angry when I question him. He has never gotten really violent, but there have been times when I was worried that he was going to hit me."

"What does he get angry about?" Mikey asked.

"It could be anything. This morning, I asked if he had brushed his teeth and he yelled at me before stomping off into the bathroom. I walked by the bathroom and he was just staring at his image in the mirror. He wasn't brushing his teeth either. He was simply staring at the mirror as if he was trying to understand what the person looking back was trying to tell him. It was really strange and it bothered me quite a bit."

"Did he brush his teeth?" Mikey asked.

"Well, when he walked back into the kitchen, I kissed him to check if he really brushed his teeth. His breath smelled so it was obvious that he hadn't brushed his teeth. I asked if did brush them and he looked at me with intense anger for a second or so. Yes, I brushed my God-damn teeth. Get off my back woman," she said.

Continuing her story, she added, "He used to go to the golf course and hit balls, but he hasn't done that for a month or so.

I ask him if he wants me to take him and he gets angry at me. He needs to find something to keep him occupied."

Mikey looked concerned as he watched his mother talk about his father. "Mom, you just relax for a while. I'll take care of Dad tonight and tomorrow."

"Thank you, Mikey," she said. "I really need a break."

After a day of having to take care of Charlie, Mikey realized that his parents needed help. He contacted the University and told them that he was forced to drop out of school for a short while due to medical problems in the family. The school accepted the withdrawal and Mikey has at least the next term free to lend a hand around the Caldwell house.

Mikey also looked at several assisted living centers in and around San Antonio. There was one specifically for older patients with dementia issues and Mikey went there to get some additional information and check it out as a possible place for them to live. He was very impressed with the facility and couldn't wait to show it to his mother.

Diane agreed to possibly move into an assisted living place after checking it out. The facility that Mikey picked out was in a beautiful location, they had assistance twenty-four hours a day and the associated restaurant seemed to be quite good. It was fairly expensive, but Charlie had his retirement income and would soon be getting disability insurance. That income, coupled with their savings would be enough to get them in and maintain their standard of living.

First thing they had to do was to get rid of a lot of items around the house. Mikey and Diane went through everything a decided they would have a garage sell to get rid of most of the items. The two had accumulated quite a bit, and it was difficult to decide what should go and what should stay. When they came to Charlie's golf clubs, Diane wanted to give them to Mikey.

"Mom, I still have the same I've had for a few years now. I only play golf every month or so and I really can't use Dad's clubs," he said.

Mikey looked at the clubs and noticed that his father still had the old three-wood that Diane gave him soon after they were married. He took it out of the bag and thought to himself, "Wow, a persimmon wood, they don't make these anymore."

Mikey put the club back in the bag and said, "Mom, you should be able to get five or six hundred dollars for these clubs and the bag in a garage sell. Go ahead and sell them," he said.

Soon, the garage and much of the back yard was full memorabilia from the Caldwell home. Mikey and Diane were in the garage during the sale when Charlie walked in. He walked around the room looking at all of the items for sale. Most of the things he picked up and looked at did not trigger any memory responses. However, there were a few items that triggered something deep in his memory that suddenly jumped to life. "Diane, I gave you this figurine on our wedding anniversary," he would say quite loudly. "Why the hell are you going to sell it?"

With each item, Diane would set it aside and say something like, "How did this get here. We don't want to sell this." She would then put it aside, where it would go right back to the "For Sale" table after Charlie forgot about it.

He stopped again when he saw his golf clubs and turned toward Diane. "Jesus!" he said quite loudly. "You cannot be thinking about selling my golf clubs."

Mikey looked up and saw his dad standing by his golf bag. Charlie took out each club and examined it carefully. He paused as he took out the three-wood. He looked like he had just found a treasure. "This really feels good," he said out loud and to himself.

After some bickering, Mikey took the golf clubs and put them back in the house. "There you go, Dad. Your golf clubs are back in the house and they're not for sale," he said.

Following the garage sale, almost everything was sold or given away. There were a few items that didn't go and Diane would simply donate them to the Goodwill Industries. She and Mikey were quite pleased with the outcome. They collected almost ten thousand dollars and made the planned move into the assisted living facility much easier.

The three went to dinner that evening and when they were eating, Charlie wanted to talk about golf. "Mikey, let's you and me go to the club tomorrow and play a round of golf," he suggested.

"Dad, it's been quite some time since I played but if you want to go, I'll go with you," Mikey said.

Early the next morning, Charlie woke Mikey up and said, "Let's go golfing, son."

The two left and drove to Pecan Valley. They walked into the pro-shop and Brett was behind the counter. "Good morning, Charlie," he said quite loud. "I see you brought your son with you today. How are you doing, Mikey?"

"Hello, Brett, I'm doing quite well. My dad talked me into playing a round of golf with him so we drove out here to see if we can get off," Mikey said.

"Sure you can. The front is open whenever you both are ready," Brett said, handing a cart key to Mikey.

Soon the two were on the first tee, looking down the beautifully groomed fairway. "Abe has done a good job with the course, hasn't he Dad?" Mikey said.

"Yeah, he's a good superintendent. You know that I brought him here when I first came, don't you?"

"I sure do, Dad. I've known Abe for as long as I can remember. He was almost like an uncle to me," Mikey added.

Mikey was the first to tee his ball down. He took out his driver and hit a fairly long ball that sliced into the right rough. "Never could get rid of the slice," he said.

Charlie walked on the tee and put his ball onto a tee. Before hitting, he turned to Mikey and said, "Son, this is as close to heaven as I can get. Playing golf with my son is perfect. However, one thing I should tell you is that I don't remember which club to hit so I will need your help. I do know that I'll use the big one here."

Hearing his dad say that he didn't know which club to hit was surprising to Mikey. He never thought about it but forgetting how far each club knocked the ball could be something that a golfer with Alzheimer's could forget. "Okay, Dad, I'll help out," he said.

Charlie stood behind the ball for a second and slowly walked up and took a perfect stance. His backswing was slow and deliberate, but as the club was heading back down, it gained speed and momentum sending the ball heading high, far and straight down the fairway.

"Great shot, Dad," said Mikey.

They drove the cart to Mikey's ball and he dribbled a three-wood down the fairway a hundred yards or so. It was still twenty yards short of Charlie's drive. Mikey hit another three-wood and almost made the green. "That's better," said Charlie.

They then stopped by Charlie's ball and Mikey made a quick measure of distance. "Dad, you drove that ball almost three hundred yards. You have about two hundred and thirty to the flag. What club do you hit at that distance?" he asked.

Charlie looked at Mikey with a questioning look on his face. "I don't have any idea. You pick the club for me," he said.

Mikey thought for a second and decided the three-wood should be enough to reach the green and handed his father the club. "Hit it right at the flag down there on the green."

Charlie repeated the motion from the tee box and took the same, perfect stance. The club came back with the same, deliberate motion and then down, making solid contact with the ball. It flew straight at the flag, going directly over the top. It landed on the far edge of the green and bounded into a hazard. "I think that one went too far," Charlie said.

"Dad, you knocked the shit out of that ball. Here, try hitting this five-wood with the same swing," Mikey said as he dropped another ball on the grass and handed his father the five-wood.

Again the same, smooth swing and the ball took off directly for the flag, landing about ten yards short and rolling another twelve.

"Dad, that was a great shot," he said. I played lots of golf with you before, but I do not remember you hitting it this well. That's unbelievable.

Charlie smiled and said, "I like this."

Mikey finished the hole making a bogey, while Charlie made his putt for a par, counting the two-shot penalty.

The next hole was a par three that measured about one hundred and eighty-five yards long. Mikey handed his father a six iron and again told him what the target line should be. Like a robot, Charlie took the same swing and sent the ball on a high flight that looked like it was going to hit the pin on the fly. The ball hit a few yards beyond the hole and backed up a foot or so.

"Mikey hit something toward the green and the two drove on. Mikey's chip was fairly close so he dragged the ball away, giving himself the putt. Charlie looked at him and asked, "Why didn't you knock the ball in the hole?"

"I gave myself that putt," Mikey said. "It was a gimme."

"What is that?" Charlie asked.

Mikey started to explain and decided to place the ball where it was and then use the putter to knock it in. "There, is that better?" he asked.

"Golf is knocking the ball into the hole," Charlie said while putting his ball straight into the hole for a birdie.

The remaining holes were about the same with Charlie hitting every green in regulation. His score would have been even better had Mikey made the right club selection for each shot. There were a couple of short pitch shots that Mikey failed to tell Charlie where to hit it and all of those were because he hit the ball too far.

Mikey tallied the scores after the round and Charlie had a sixty-eight. Mikey was a bit embarrassed about telling father that he shot eighty-eight. "That's good, Mikey. I had a really good time. Let's play again tomorrow," Charlie suggested.

"Okay, let's first see if Mom has anything going on. If she doesn't we'll certainly come back out and play."

The next day, the arrived at the course about the same time and Bobby Holiday was there practicing. As they were on the tee box, Bobby came up and asked to join them. Mikey looked at Charlie who said, "Sure, you can play with us."

Bobby saw that they were playing from the middle tees and asked if they wanted to play from the back as that was where he normally played from.

Mikey said that they preferred to play from the white tees but Charlie intervened and said, "Sure, we can play from the back tees if you want."

Mikey was again first to play and hit his high, slicing drive about two hundred yards. Charlie was going to be next but asked Bobby to tee off first.

Bobby was a fairly big and healthy young man and could hit the ball into the next county. He hit a high drive that seemed to carry forever but didn't have any forward roll as it landed in the rough. "Nice shot," said Mikey.

Charlie then teed his ball up from the back tees and like yesterday, took his slow and deliberate back swing. Again the ball took off on a low trajectory, heading straight for the center of the fairway. It stopped a few yards farther than Bobby's high ball.

"Damn, that was huge," said Bobby.

Charlie didn't say anything. He just smiled.

Like yesterday, Mikey moved the ball down the fairway and closer to the green each time. Bobby hit an iron and stopped just short of the green.

Charlie looked at his ball and wondered what to hit. He grabbed his driver but Mikey stepped in. "Dad, you don't want this club," he said taking the driver from Charlie's hands. "I have you at two hundred and sixty yards. Here, hit this," he said handing his father the three-wood.

Like yesterday, Charlie's ball headed straight for the green, landing just short and bouncing onto the surface. The ball rolled toward the pin, stopping just inches from the cup.

"Holy-mackerel," said Bobby. "That was the best two shots I've ever seen on this hole. Nice eagle, Mister Caldwell."

When they reached the green, Bobby walked up and saw that Charlie was only a foot away from the hole. He knocked the ball back to Charlie.

Mikey started to say something but Charlie beat him to it. "Son," he said, addressing Bobby. "We must knock every ball into the hole. We don't do these... what do you call them, Mikey?"

"Gimme's, Dad," said Mikey.

"Yeah, we don't do gimme's here," said Charlie.

Bobby chipped up and two-putted for his par and then put Charlie's ball back where it was.

Charlie tapped in for an eagle.

The round today was much like the one from yesterday. Mikey was in the middle eighties, Bobby was at even par and Charlie shot a smooth sixty-five. It would have been better but Mikey didn't select the right club on a couple of shots and they ended up a bit short.

"That's the best round I've ever seen out here," said Bobby after the round and the three were in the restaurant having a coke. "You're hitting the ball great."

Abe heard that Charlie and Mikey were at the club and walked into the restaurant and joined them.

"Hey, Charlie," Abe said. "It's been quite some time since you've been back. I thought you were giving up the game."

"Giving up the game," said Bobby. "This guy just shot the easiest sixty-five I've ever witnessed. He had an eagle and five birdies."

"Wow," Abe replied. "That's the ole 'All or Nothing' dude I used to caddie for, huh?"

Charlie smiled at Abe. "All or Nothing, I remember that. They used to call me that when we were playing, huh."

"You bet," said Abe. "You were known as the 'All or Nothing' dude from Nowhere, Texas."

After finishing their cokes, Mikey and Charlie headed back home while Abe did a little research. He heard of a group of ex-golfers that formed a group in South Texas. They played different courses and competed for small cash prizes. He found out where the group was located and discovered their next tournament was here in San Antonio at the Dominion. He called the office of the Southern Texas Senior PGA and got Charlie entered.

Afterwards, Abe called Mikey and told him what he'd done. Mikey was hesitant as he wasn't sure if his father could actually play competitive golf. "Are you going to caddie for him?" asked Mikey.

"I don't know if I could carry the clubs around for eighteen holes, dude. Maybe I could, but I think he would be more comfortable with you," replied Abe. "He seems to enjoy it more so you go ahead and caddie for him. I think everyone rides so you really won't have to carry the bag."

The following Monday was the first round and Charlie was interested in playing at the Dominion but wasn't overly thrilled. "Why can't you play too, Mikey?" he asked.

"Dad, this is a senior tournament and I'm not close to being a senior. This is your tournament. I'll drive the cart for you and tell you which clubs to hit and where to aim them at. The rest is up to you."

"Okay," replied Charlie.

"I'm just along to see some great golf," added Abe.

The tournament was a shotgun start and Abe's group started on number four. This hole was a short, par-four and didn't require a driver off the tee. Mikey handed Charlie a three-wood and told him to hit it right over the top of the tree next to the right side of the fairway. Charlie was lined up perfectly and followed Mikey's direction to a tee. His ball ended up a mere ninety yards from the green.

The second shot was pretty straight forward but the distance was right between the sand wedge and pitching wedge. Mikey handed the sand wedge to Charlie and instructed him to land it near the middle of the green. As instructed the ball took off high and landed ten feet to the right of the flag but in the middle of the green.

"Perfect, Dad," said Mikey.

Charlie missed the putt but having a par on the starting hole of a tournament was not considered to be bad at all.

The sixth hole was a challenging but short par four. It was only three hundred and ten yards and most golfers elected to hit an iron then have a wedge to the green for an easy birdie.

Mikey handed a five-iron to Charlie and instructed him to hit it to the middle of the fairway. Charlie was ready to hit but stopped and backed up. "Mikey, I can get reach this hole with the big one. Why don't you want to use it?"

"Dad, an iron will take most of the trouble out of play. If you miss it short and right, you will be in some heavy and deep bunkers. I think the five-iron is right."

"Let me try the big club," asked Charlie.

"Okay, use the big one but remember, I told you hitting the driver here could get you in trouble."

Charlie stood behind the teed up ball and appeared to be studying the shot. He then walked up and took the slow, deliberate swing as he used with his previous tee shot. The ball took off on a higher trajectory and was heading straight for the green. It looked like it was falling out of the air and would land in the greenside bunker. Fortunately, it carried the bunker and with one bounce was on the green heading for the cup. It stopped a few feet short of the hole.

Charlie smiled at Mikey and said, "I knew I could do it."

Abe had watched this shot and right after Charlie sent the ball flying, Abe said, "Mikey, let me introduce you to All or Nothing!"

As the group was walking off the green, Mikey looked at Abe and winked. "Great shot, huh?"

"He used to do it all the time," said Abe. "Often it was 'All' but frequently it was also 'Nothing'."

Mikey just smiled as he put the putter into the bag.

The eagle on number six, coupled with three other birdies, gave Charlie a five-under sixty-six and he was leading the other golfers by four shots after the first day.

The second day of this two day event saw Charlie repeating his performance. He ended up with a one hundred and thirty-three for the two day event. First prize was $1,450 but he also won a skin for his eagle on number six, which gave him a total cash prize of over $2,000.

When Mikey and Charlie got home that afternoon after winning the golf tournament, Diane was at the door waiting. "Well, how did it go, Charlie?" she asked.

Charlie looked at his wife with a puzzled look. "How did what go?"

"The golf tournament, silly, how did you play today?"

"I wasn't in a tournament. I just played golf with some friends," Charlie said, still not sure exactly what his wife was talking about.

"Well, what was your score?" she asked, knowing that he was in the lead after the first day.

Charlie thought long and hard for a moment before answering, "Hell, I don't remember. Mikey, did you keep my score?"

"Yes, Dad, you shot sixty-six today and won the tournament by eight shots," Mikey said excitingly. "Better yet, Mom, he made an eagle on a hole and that was good for a six hundred dollar skin!"

"Well, how about that?" she said. "I know two men who need to take me out to dinner."

"I'm hungry," said Charlie. "What's for dinner?"

"Just a moment, I'll grab my purse and we'll go somewhere and have dinner," she said.

Charlie entered several other small, professional tournaments in the Southern Texas area, winning each one by a substantial number. During one of the tournaments, a couple of golfers in the group suggested that Charlie try to qualify for the Senior Open. The local qualifying was going to be held at Brackenridge Golf Course in San Antonio and the top winner was guaranteed entry and the second person would be listed as an alternate entry.

Mikey got all the details and entered his dad into the qualifying. They played a practice round at Brackenridge but the practice round was for Mikey to understand the course and distances. This would allow him to better club Charlie. If he knew the distance, he should be able to give Charlie the correct club to hit. If done correctly, it should be good for five or six birdies a round.

The date of the qualifying was at hand and Charlie and Mikey were waiting on the tee at Brackenridge when Charlie's name was called. As usual, Charlie hit the ball straight down the middle of the fairway and Mikey gave him the perfect club for the second shot. This led to an easy birdie and after the front side; Charlie was coasting to an easy five-under par. The back had a couple of reachable par-fives and Charlie hit one of them in two, making an eagle. When he finished, Charlie was at the scorer's table while Mikey was getting something to drink. Thinking he had plenty of time to review the scores with his father, he was not in a big hurry.

The official scorer noticed a smudged number on Charlie's card and had a difficult time reading the number. "Charlie, what did you score on number thirteen?" he asked.

"Hell, I don't know," replied Charlie. "It's whatever is on the card."

The scorer was caught by surprise. "Charlie, you know the rules say that the player must be responsible for his score. There are no exceptions to this rule. I cannot read the card for sure. It looks like it could be a three or maybe a five. Which is it?" he asked again.

Charlie looked at the scorer again and said, "Look, I told you I don't remember what I made. Put me down for anything, I don't care. I was just playing golf and don't need some son-of-a-bitch to be yelling at me."

The official seemed to be upset. "Sir, you have signed your card but cannot verify your scores. Rule Six specifically states that the player must be able to verify his score as posted on the score card. You cannot verify this, so I'm sorry to say, you must be disqualified."

About this time, Mikey walked up and saw that his father was upset. "What's the matter, Dad?" he asked.

"This son-of-a-bitch just told me that I was disqualified because I couldn't remember my score on one of the holes," Charlie replied barely trying to hold back his anger.

"What hole? Sir, I know the score of every hole. What hole do you have in question?" Mikey asked.

"Sir, it really doesn't make any difference now. Your father has officially been disqualified from this event. Rule Six in the USGA Rules of Golf specifically states that the golfer must be able to verify his score on any holes played. We asked him to verify his score for number thirteen several times, but he says he doesn't remember. We're very sorry, but we must follow the rules as stated," replied the official.

Mikey leaned over and at a low whisper, said, "Sir, my father has Alzheimer's and he has trouble remembering what he did a few minutes ago. Trying to get him to remember that he made an eagle on number thirteen would be impossible. Please reverse your decision," Mikey pleaded.

"The only thing I can do for you is to bring this matter up in front of the four other officials we have at this event. If they rule to overturn my ruling, then your father's score will count. If not, then my ruling will have to stand."

"The question is whether he made a three or a five on the par-five   , thirteenth. If you just give him a five, he'll still be way ahead of the pack. Can you do this?" Mikey asked.

"No, Sir," responded the official. "I cannot do this. Besides, the rule infraction is not what he made on a particular hole, but him not being able to be responsible for his score."

Mikey was upset, but paused before going off on the official. "When will you meet with the other officials?" Mikey asked.

"I'm calling them in now. When they get here, we will have a closed session and announce our ruling immediately after we adjourn."

The other officials came and the four of them went into a private office and the scorer had Charlie's card with him. After ten minutes, they returned and the three that came in from the course immediately went back out, not saying anything before leaving.

The lead official walked up to Mikey and Charlie and told them that his ruling would stand. He was terribly sorry but he was not allowed to circumvent an official rule.

Charlie didn't seem to care and wanted to go get something at his favorite place to eat, "Whataburger." Mikey on the other hand, was beyond words. "Dad, I'm sorry. I should have stayed with you but I didn't think the scoring would be so quick. It's my fault," said Mikey.

"Hell, Mikey, don't worry about it. It was just another golf tournament and there are plenty more. Let's go eat," said Charlie.

"Dad, it's just not right," said Mikey. "You had the lowest score and should not have been penalized for simply not remembering what it was. This isn't right."

As the two walked toward the parking area, one of the golfers that played in the group with Charlie stopped them. He simply wanted to congratulate Charlie on his stellar play. "That was the very best golf I've ever seen today, Charlie. That even includes all the tournaments on television. You certainly deserve a shot at winning the Senior Open. You are one hell of a golfer."

"I guess it was Okay," said Charlie. "I don't remember very much though. We're going to get a Whataburger now."

Mikey spoke up and informed the golfer that Charlie had been disqualified for not being able to recall his score. "The scorer asked Charlie to verify the score for the par five, number thirteen. Dad told him that he didn't remember and that led to the scorer invoking Rule Number Six which governs the player's responsibilities. We appealed the ruling but their committee met on it and they did not change the ruling. I guess we will have to wait until next year," Mikey said.

"That is total horseshit," said the golfer. He called the other player in the group over and this was the one that smudged the number on the card. "Bob, they disqualified Charlie for not being able to remember what he made on number thirteen. Do you believe that?"

"I was the scorer and he hit a perfect second shot. Charlie then made a ten-foot eagle putt. I messed up the holes and accidentally first wrote a five on the card. Charlie made a great three on that hole and I'll go in and straighten this out," he said making a dash to the scorer's area.

He came back a few minutes later and was told that the number on the card really didn't matter. The simple fact that Charlie couldn't be responsible for all of his scores was the issue. "They refused to even listen to me," he said. "This is crap and I'll raise the issue to someone who will listen."

Mikey thanked them for anything they could do but had basically written it off. He grabbed his dad and they headed off to get a Whataburger.

The golfer that recorded Charlie's scores contacted one of the local television stations that had a camera crew on site. He located the reporter that was doing the story and passed on the incident concerning Charlie. The cameraman recorded the interview and it made the evening news. The crew tried to find Charlie so they could get the information from the source, but Charlie and Mikey were long gone to Whataburger.

The next day, the story made the National News and the entire country soon knew about Charlie and his problem with the United States Golf Association. The report also said that Charlie was affected with early stages of Alzheimer's and that only added fuel to the fire.

On Sunday afternoon, the phone rang at the Caldwell's and it was the USGA calling. They were informed about Charlie's plight during the qualifying round and wanted to provide Charlie with an exemption. This meant that Charlie would be entered into the tournament. The person that came in second, five shots behind Charlie would also qualify. The USGA took full responsibility for this situation and would provide airline tickets for both Charlie and his caddie. However, they would have to fly on Monday since there were no flights that would get them into Rochester on Sunday.

Diane took the call and related the story to both Mikey and Charlie. Mikey was extremely happy but Charlie didn't let on if he really cared.

"Dad," Mikey said. "We're going to play in the Senior Open next week. What do you think about that?"

"Okay, Mikey," Charlie replied as he was focused on the television show he was watching.

"Mom, this is great. Dad has a chance to really show the world that simply being diagnosed with early stages of Alzheimer's doesn't mean it's the end of the world. Dad will show them that they can still accomplish great things," Mikey said excitingly.

"Well, Mikey, just make sure that you are doing this for Charlie and that you will take his best interest in heart. I don't want to see him suffer needlessly by playing in a high profile and high stress golf tournament," Diane added.

"Hell Mom, Dad doesn't have any idea what kind of tournament he's playing or who he's playing with. Playing with Tom Watson or Jack Nicklaus would be nothing more than playing with one of the locals from the club."

"That's true," she added.

The tournament was going to be held at Oak Hill Country Club in Rochester, New York. Mikey had to contact the travel agent that was provided by the USGA. Mikey tried to get his mother to go with them but Diane said she would prefer not to go. She said she would watch on television.

Mikey thought about arriving late and having only two practice rounds. After talking with Diane, they both agreed that it was actually good to limit Charlie's time away from home as much as possible. Besides, Charlie really didn't need several practice rounds on the course. One would be plenty as long as Mikey gave him the right club and told him where to hit it.

Within minutes, Mikey had reservations for a Monday flight to Rochester. They would leave San Antonio around ten in the morning and arrive in Rochester around six in the early evening. The tournament committee already had reservations in one of the hotels so Mikey didn't have to do anything there.

He wanted to be able to travel around so he also took advantage of the free rental cars offered to the players. He and

Charlie would have a new Buick to take them to and from the golf course.

Chapter Eight

Their room at the DoubleTree was quite nice. It was on the third floor and Mikey was certainly glad that the USGA blocked so many rooms to be used for the tournament. Unlike most of the professionals playing in the tournament, Charlie and Mikey were on an extremely limited budget and the accommodations at the DoubleTree were much better than they expected. As they were checking in, lots of people were moving around the lobby area and most looked like they just walked in from the golf course. Since most just came in from a Monday practice round, they were still wearing their Nike, Titleist or TaylorMade hats and it seemed that everyone knew everyone else.

It was too late in the afternoon to go out to Oak Hill Country Club so Mikey and Charlie stayed in the room and watched television. Later, they went downstairs and walked over to Charlie's second favorite place to eat, McDonalds.

After dinner, they walked back to the room and watched a bit more television. Before falling asleep, Mikey double-checked the door to ensure it was locked and just to make sure nothing happened, he hung a small bell from the door knob. If Charlie awakened during the night and tried to walk out of the room, he would have to get past the two locks and this was an extremely difficult task for Charlie. However, just to make sure, the bell would sound if he was somehow successful.

During breakfast on Monday morning, Mikey watched golf professional, Nick Price go through the buffet line, while having a conversation with Greg Norman who was on the other side of the serving line. They were discussing problems with their flights into Rochester on Sunday.

Meanwhile, Charlie was oblivious to what was happening around him. He was totally focused on the waffle he had in front of him. He cut it into small pieces and began eating it without syrup. "Mikey, do we have any of the stuff that makes these things taste real good?" he asked.

Not remembering the names of common objects is very common in people suffering from Alzheimer's and Charlie used common words like 'stuff' and 'things' more and more frequently. "Yes Dad, we have some syrup for your waffle right here," he said as he handed Charlie the glass syrup dispenser.

Charlie struggled with sliding the bar open while trying to pour syrup on the waffles. It was obvious that he forgot how to work the contraption and was becoming a bit frustrated. "God-damn thing is broken," Charlie said out loud, slamming the bottle on the table. Luckily, it didn't break.

Mikey noticed the trouble his dad was having and intervened when Charlie slammed the bottle down. "Here Dad, let me help," said Mikey as he took the container from the table and poured a generous amount of the sweet stuff on Charlie's things. Hoping to make his father feel a bit better, he added, "They sure make these bottles hard to use, huh?"

A simple grunt of approval was all that came from Charlie as he dug into his cut up waffles.

After eating breakfast, Charlie and Mikey went back to their room to get ready for their scheduled 11:30am practice round. Leaving the hotel at 9:30am gave them plenty of time to check out the locker rooms, practice area, and putting green before heading out.

Charlie was very excited about playing golf on a new golf course and with new people. When Mikey suggested it was time to leave, Charlie was out of the door. However, when he entered the hallway, he couldn't remember which way to go to find the elevator.

"Which way do we go to catch the thing that takes us to the ground?" he asked with a questioning look on his face.

"Let's go this way," Mikey said, pointing to the hallway to the left. "I think the elevator is down here."

They were soon in the car, taking the short, ten-minute drive to Oak Hills Country Club. Stopping at the entrance to the club house grounds, a security guard stopped the two. It was obvious the guard didn't recognize them. "Sir, this entrance is for players only."

"I'm Mikey Caldwell and this is Charlie Caldwell. He's my father and is playing in the tournament."

After showing identification and the guard checking the list, the two were waved through. They drove slowly through the massive oak trees and soon arrived at the steps of a large and beautiful club house. "This is it, Dad. We're finally here. Do you want to go play some golf?" he asked.

Charlie was still looking at the entrance way in wonderment of the huge trees. "Okay, Mikey, let's play some golf."

Two attendants quickly ran up to the car and opened both doors. "Welcome to Oak Hills. May we get your golf clubs?" one of the attendants asked.

Mikey was already out of the car and walking toward the trunk when he replied, "Sure, you can get the clubs." He opened the trunk and the attendant was a bit surprised to see an older golf bag that was not branded with one of the standard golf company's logos such as Titleist, Callaway, or Ping.

As he lifted the bag and took it out of the trunk, the attendant couldn't help but notice that the golf clubs were an older set of McGregor irons and a mix-match of woods. Normally, the attendants used a towel to clean off the clubs but the condition of this set of clubs caused him to think otherwise.

Mikey handed the keys to the rental car to one of the attendants while the other attendant placed Charlie's set of clubs next to other bags that were much larger, marked with some sort of logo and had the name of the golfer embroidered on the side. Mikey then handed each a couple of dollars as a tip before he took Charlie into the locker room.

Another attendant was at the door of the locker room and failed to recognize Charlie and Mikey as one of the golfers. "Sir, I'm sorry but this is for players only."

Charlie said, "I play golf."

The locker room attendant smiled and started to say something when Mikey jumped in. "This is Charlie Caldwell and he's playing in the tournament. I'm his son and his caddie and I believe the USGA officials made an exception to the rule of players only and are allowing me in the clubhouse to help my father."

The attendant checked his list and found Charlie's name. "I have Mister Caldwell on the list but do not have anything about allowing his caddie into the locker room."

"But, I was told that they made an exception for us. I'm not only his caddie, I'm also his son. Can you please…" he was starting to ask when the door opened as Jay Haas and another golfer walked out of the locker room. "Sir, as I was saying the USGA made an exception for us and if you would check it out, you will find that we should have authorization to both enter the locker room."

"I'll be glad to check but can't leave the area until someone comes to relieve me. If you both would wait outside, I'll come and get you when I get confirmation."

Mikey was getting upset but was not surprised when he learned that the USGA failed to follow up on something they said would happen. Charlie's entry and performance during the qualifying tournament created lots of controversy and many of the senior USGA folks didn't approve of the exception offered to Charlie. "OKAY, forget about it right now. All we need to do is to change shoes. Can we leave the shoes here while we go out and play a practice round?" Mikey asked.

"Mister Caldwell can go in. He can leave the shoes there and change clothes if necessary. He cannot leave his shoes here," replied the attendant.

Mikey got close to the attendant's face and whispered, "My father has Alzheimer's and I cannot leave him alone. The USGA told me that they were making arrangements where I could be with him at all times. It seems they may have missed the locker room portion, so we'll just go out and hit some balls before he plays the practice round today. Please try to get this squared away for tomorrow, Okay? In the meantime, we'll put his street shoes in the bag."

"I'll do what I can. Your father can put on his golf shoes and leave the other shoes here. I'll ensure they get placed in his locker," replied the attendant.

"Thank you," said Mikey as he turned to have Charlie change into his golf shoes.

"Dad, put your golf shoes on and leave your regular shoes here. This man will put them inside the locker room for us."

"Okay," replied Charlie.

They were almost at the door of the clubhouse when the attendant caught up with them. "Excuse me, I think you will need this to get on the range," he said, handing Mikey the clip-on badge that identified Charlie as a player. "It was on the locker."

"Okay, thanks! I think we would have had a hard time getting on the range, let alone the actual course without this. Thanks again," replied Mikey.

Mikey placed the clip-on badge on Charlie's collar and then picked up the clubs. They went to the driving range that was now full of golfers hitting shot after shot down range. The guard at the range noticed Charlie's badge and ushered them both onto the range area.

Mikey found an open spot between Isao Aoki and another professional golfer that he didn't recognize. "Charlie, let's go over here and hit some balls," he said, pointing to the empty spot.

"Okay," replied Charlie.

As soon as they were at the open spot, another attendant brought a bucket of new Titleist golf balls. Charlie, let out a small smile when he saw all the balls. "Mikey, these are brand-new golf balls," he said.

"Yeah Dad, that's what they use here. This is not like the driving range at Pecan Valley, is it?"

"No, they have brand new balls here," added Charlie.

Mikey handed his father a pitching wedge and said, "Here Dad, hit a few wedges just to warm up."

Charlie was still focused on seeing so many brand new golf balls as a took the wedge from Mikey. He turned toward Isao Aoki and noticed that he also had new golf balls for practicing. "Hey fella," he said loudly. "You got new balls too. This is amazing, huh"

Aoki looked up and smiled slightly at Charlie before returning his focus on trying to hit the ball with the precision he had in his former days.

Charlie turned back around where he saw Mikey was waiting for him. "Okay," replied Charlie, as he took his classic grip on the wedge.

"Dad, see how close you can come to hitting the one hundred hard sign," said Mikey.

Using the same, smooth and easy-looking swing each time, Charlie put ball after ball within feet of the hundred yard sign. He actually hit the sign with two shots and Mikey watched intently as his father went through his warm-up routine.

Handing his father a nine-iron, he said, "Dad, here's the nine. How about hitting these about twenty yards over the sign?"

"Okay," replied Charlie as he took the same swing as before. Again, ball after ball flew directly over the one hundred yard sign and each stopped within mere feet of the others. "Nice shot group, Dad," Mikey said giving positive feedback to his father.

Mikey repeated this drill with different clubs, and eventually worked his way to the driver. Charlie was using an older Titleist driver and its head was much smaller than drivers that the other players were using. Though it was a much older club, Charlie was hitting it in the center of the club face, driving the ball well down the range. Shot after shot, the ball rocketed off the tee with a very slight draw.

Mikey didn't notice the person that came up behind. "Hello, Mister Caldwell, my name is Jay Bruce and I'm the Titleist representative here. I noticed that your father is using an older set of woods. Would you be interested in trying out one of our new line of Titleist Woods?"

"Thank you sir, but we really can't afford to buy new clubs at this time," replied Mikey.

"Oh, there's no cost. The only thing we ask is that you use the head-covers that come with the club. Besides the driver, it looks like you have a three-wood and five-wood in the bag. Is that correct?" Jay asked.

"Yes, that is what we have," replied Mikey.

"Do you know if that shaft is a regular or stiff shaft?"

Mikey looked at the Titleist rep with a questioning look on his face. "I have no idea. As far as I know, it is the same shaft that came with the original club," replied Mikey.

The Titleist rep looked a bit surprised. "Okay, let's see what we can do to determine the best shaft for your father. With his swing and distance based upon the older Titleist driver he's using, I think we'll try a shaft that is in between the regular and stiff shaft. I'll have these clubs in just a few minutes."

"Okay, but I will tell you that my dad doesn't react very well to changes. You bring me the clubs and I'll work something out to see if we can get him to try them. If we just tell him that we have new clubs for him to use, he'll not be too receptive to the idea."

"Okay, I'll let you handle that part of it. Just a minute and we'll have some new clubs for you," said Jay as he turned and hurried to his equipment van.

Within a few minutes, he was back with three clubs in a Titleist bag. He handed the bag to Mikey and said, "See if he likes these and we've also thrown in a staff bag."

"Okay, I'll see what he thinks of the new clubs," Mikey said as he picked up the bag and turned toward Charlie. "Hey Dad, I found these new clubs over here in this golf bag and they said we could have them. How about trying them to see if you can gain any distance?"

"Okay," replied Charlie as he set the older driver down. "This is brand new, isn't it?" Charlie asked.

"Yes, it's brand new. Try hitting a few balls with it."

Charlie teed up a ball and again took the same, exact swing. The ball flew off the tee with the same trajectory as the other driver. Because of the improvements in club design, the ball must have come off the club much faster as it carried another twenty or thirty yards past the other drives hit with the older driver.

He hit another drive and it went even farther than the first. Mikey looked back at Jay Bruce and Jay was smiling with an ear-to-ear grin. "Nice shot," he yelled out.

Mikey was totally surprised when Charlie handed the club back to Mikey. "What's wrong with the club, Dad? You hit that last ball much farther than with the other driver."

"Mikey, Diane bought me these clubs and I've gotten used to hitting them. Tell the person to give them to one of the other golfers here. Look, there are lots of golfers and I bet one of them can use a new driver. I'll stay with the clubs that Diane gave me."

Mikey knew that it would be futile to try to convince his father otherwise so he took the three clubs and carried them back to Jay Bruce. "Mister Bruce, my father really likes the clubs but wants to use his clubs as Mom bought them for him. It wouldn't do any good for me to continue to argue with him."

"Okay, but do you realize that he gained at least thirty yards on his tee shot?"

"Yes, I saw it too. However, my dad has made up his mind and believe me there's nothing we can do to change it at this point," replied Mikey.

"Alright then, please keep us in mind if and when he wants to upgrade," replied Jay as he took the clubs back. He stopped and walked back to Mikey. "Does your father use Titleist balls?" he asked.

"Yeah, we have a couple of sleeves. We were going to pocket a few of these balls on the range though."

"You don't have to do that. I'll make sure that two dozen balls are in your dad's locker room tonight."

"That's super. Thanks, Jay," Mikey said as he shook the rep's hand.

Charlie stayed with the old clubs and now hit a dozen or so sand wedges as he completed his warm-up routine.

"Okay, Dad. Let's go putt a few before we tee off."

"Okay," replied Charlie.

The two walked through the crowd of people and the fans were asking for autographs. No one recognized Charlie as one of the players so few people wanted his autograph. He did sign one or two on the way to the putting green. His signature was a scratchy scribble that was simply "Charlie." One fan asked Charlie to sign a cap, which Charlie did. "I just signed that fella's cap," he said to Mikey with a surprised look on his face.

When they reached the practice green, Mikey reached in the bag and pulled out Charlie's old Arnold Palmer blade putter. It was old but it was like gold when it was in Charlie's hands. He brought it straight back, had a very slight pause and he then took it straight through the ball. He handed the putter to Charlie and then pulled out one of the two sleeves of new golf balls. "Here Dad, let's use new balls today."

"Okay," replied Charlie.

They practiced from three feet, five feet and fifteen feet. Charlie was making most of the putts and only missed putts from the fifteen feet mark.

It was now time to go to the tee, so Mikey grabbed the bag and placed the putter in it before guiding Charlie through the crowd and to the number one tee box. The other player that was assigned the same tee time was another qualifier. They were only a two-some so it would be a long, practice round.

They waited until the group in front was well out of range and the other golfer hit the first shot, missing the fairway on the right. Charlie then got up and just like on the range, the ball flew on a low trajectory with a very slight draw. It landed in the middle of the fairway and rolled another twenty or thirty yards. The small crowd around the first tee clapped and Charlie smiled back at them.

Charlie played the practice round without any problems and Mikey took notes on each hole. He was picking out landing spots and trying to notice the main slopes around each green. All in all, it was a good practice round, Charlie got to play a round of golf on a beautiful course and Mikey was able to capture some valuable distance information.

When they finished the round, Mikey and Charlie were walking through the crowd of golf fans toward the club house. The plan was to change shoes, leave the clubs in club storage and then go to a restaurant in the Rochester area.

Just before they entered the club house, Mikey heard someone call out, "Charlie!" Charlie stopped and looked at where he thought the sound had come from. He saw the man walking quickly toward them. It was Abe.

Charlie immediately recognized his best friend. "Hey, Abe," he called out. "Did Diane come with you?"

"Nah, Charlie, Diane couldn't make it, so I just decided to get on a plane and come and watch. This should be quite a show," Abe added

"Abe, do you want to play golf with us today?" Charlie asked.

Mikey broke in, "Dad, we've already played golf today. We're not going to play any more golf today. We are going to change your shoes and then go get something to eat. Let's invite Abe to join us for dinner,"

Charlie looked at Mikey with a questioning look, "Dinner? Are we going to Whataburger?" Charlie asked.

"No, we're going to Milts," replied Mikey. "You know, we talked about it on the drive here this morning."

Abe jumped in. "I don't know where Milts is but I'll join you. My rental car is in the public parking lot so it will take me longer to get to my car than it will take you. I'll find the place and join you when I get there."

"Okay, see you soon," replied Mikey. Charlie didn't say anything.

The attendant saw Mikey and Charlie walk up and immediately opened the door to the locker room. "Afternoon, Mister Caldwell. We got confirmation of the exception and you'll be fine for the rest of the week."

Mikey replied with a "Thank you" as he followed Charlie into the locker room. Charlie's sat down on the bench and untied his golf shoes. Leaning over, he reached for his dress shoes and noticed that each had a lustrous shine on them. "Mikey, they shined my shoes." Charlie turned to another golf pro that was putting on a dress shirt a couple of lockers away and said proudly, "I've got shined shoes!"

The pro took the comment in stride and said, "Yes, they do a good job at this club."

"Shined shoes… shined shoes." Charlie kept repeating it as he changed shoes.

Within minutes, Charlie had changed his shoes and Mikey had the clubs put away. "Let's go get some dinner," Mikey said.

"Okay," replied Charlie, still looking at his shined shoes.

They arrived at Milt's Family Diner and were already seated when Abe walked in. He saw Mikey signaling and walked over and sat down in the booth next to Charlie.

Charlie looked at him and said, "Hello, my name is Charlie Caldwell. What is your name?"

Abe looked surprised but took it in stride and replied, "Hello Charlie. My name is Abe and I used to be your caddie."

Charlie smiled with a huge grin, "I remember you now. Abe do you know Mikey? He is my caddie now. He's a really good caddie, too."

"Yes, I know. I saw you and Mikey playing golf today and I agree with you, Mikey is a great caddie."

The three made small conversation through dinner and as Charlie was drinking his after dinner coffee, Abe looked at Mikey. "Mikey, I know it is just you and Charlie here this week. You can't leave him so I'm offering my services. If you need me to watch Charlie for a few minutes or hours, let me know. I'm staying at the Howard Johnson Motel out by the airport."

"Well thank you very much, Abe. I wish we could get you into the hotel where we're staying but I would imagine that they are full."

"That's Okay," replied Abe. "The place I'm staying in is a hell of a lot cheaper than the DoubleTree. It's clean and kind of quiet, too."

"We're planning to go off early tomorrow morning," said Mikey. "If you want to join us, you will need to be there by 7am."

"I ain't got anywhere else to go," replied Abe. "I'll be there."

Finally, it was time to head back to the DoubleTree so Abe said, "Charlie, good luck in the tournament. Remember, I'm here with you and will follow you around the course tomorrow."

"Okay," replied Charlie.

As they were driving back to the DoubleTree, Charlie asked, "Mikey, who was that fellow that had dinner with us? I think I know him."

"Just a friend, Dad," said Mikey.

Charlie was tired and went to bed right after taking a shower. Mikey watched a little TV and then turned out the light. He remembered to chain the lock to the door and attach the bell so Charlie couldn't get up and slip outside during the middle of the night.

As usual, Charlie was up early. He was in the bathroom and was talking to himself. Mikey got up, walked to the bathroom to find Charlie leaning over the sink and mumbling to himself. It looked like he was trying to figure out where he left his toothbrush.

"Dad, what's going on in here?" Mikey asked.

"I can't find the God-damn toothbrush. I looked in the thing we put it in but it's not there. Where did you hide it?" he asked with lots of anger in his tone.

"Dad, it's right there in the glass with the toothpaste and my toothbrush," Mikey replied as he reached for it to hand it to Charlie.

"I see the God-damn thing. It wasn't there just a minute ago, dammit."

"That's Okay, Dad. It was hard to find but you found it," Mikey replied trying to soothe his father.

"Well quit hiding it Mikey. My memory is not very good anymore and when you hide things from me, it makes me mad as hell."

Mikey took the toothbrush and put a good amount of toothpaste on the bristles. "Here Dad, brush your teeth and after I brush mine, we will go get some pancakes."

The sudden thought of pancakes turned Charlie around. "Pancakes?" replied Charlie. "We can get pancakes here, really?"

"Sure can. They have blueberry pancakes in the restaurant downstairs. I guess you didn't see them yesterday, but we'll make sure you see them today."

Both completed their morning chores and went downstairs to the empty restaurant. Like yesterday, there was a full buffet. It was just after six in the morning and the other golfers were still sleeping, so they had the entire restaurant to themselves.

Mikey led Charlie to the pancakes and helped him put three, fluffy blueberry pancakes on his plate. "Here you go, Dad. Let's put some maple syrup on them now" Mikey said as he put a generous helping of maple syrup on Charlie's pancakes.

"Okay," replied Charlie as he took the plate and walked to the first booth he came to. Mikey finished getting his breakfast plate loaded and joined his father.

"How are the pancakes, Dad?" he asked.

"They are pretty good. I like pancakes," replied Charlie.

"Yes, I know you do."

After breakfast, Mikey decided to head to the course and get an early round in. As planned, they were going to play on Wednesday then do something in the afternoon.

It was just before 7am when they arrived and they were the first ones there. They dropped the car off with the one attendant that was available and walked into the locker room. Charlie's shoes were outside of his locker and like the shoes from yesterday, these were cleaned and shined.

"Dad, look here. Your golf shoes are shined too!" Mikey said.

Charlie smiled softly and said, "Okay."

They went to the range and were the only golfers on the range when the gates were opened. About ten or twelve fans took seats behind the range, waiting until the big name professionals arrived. They wanted to make sure they had the best seats so they arrived early. They were talking about the major players and reviewing their tee times for the day and Mikey could hear the muffled conversations. He also heard the conversation concerning the person hitting balls. "Who is that?" one fan asked to the others.

"I don't recognize him but I think that is the golfer with Alzheimer's. I believe his name is Charlie Caldwell from Texas," replied the other fan.

100

"Oh yes, that's got to be him. Frank was telling us about the golfer yesterday that had the old bag with the mixed clubs. They said he was the golfer that had Alzheimer's," another fan in the group replied.

"Alzheimer's... how can he have Alzheimer's and play golf with that disease. Doesn't it totally incapacitate you?" another fan asked.

"No, not from what I understand. First, you have memory loss and then eventually, you'll forget how to do basic things. I guess this person is not that far along or maybe golf is like riding a bike, you just don't seem to forget how to do it."

"I heard that he was disqualified at the qualifier in Texas but the USGA made an exception and let him play without fully qualifying," another fan replied.

"Well, if you ask me that is a crock of shit. If you're disqualified, it doesn't really matter why. You're still disqualified. It really isn't fair to all the other golfers that barely missed qualifying, especially when they obeyed the rules," replied the other fan.

Mikey had heard enough. He handed his father another club and said, "Dad, here's a three iron. See if you can hit the 200 yard sign."

"Okay," replied Charlie.

Charlie began hitting shots that were all real close to the 200 yard sign. Watching the first few shots, Mikey turned and walked back to the fans that were talking earlier. "Hello guys. My name is Mikey Caldwell and Charlie's my father. He does have Alzheimer's and every single day brings us different obstacles. Some are easy and almost funny at times. However, others are very serious and almost impossible to deal with. Your observation with the golf clubs is correct. Dad has an old bag with a mixed set of clubs. He was offered a new set of Titleist clubs yesterday but turned the offer down because his wife, my mother bought these clubs for him some time ago."

"That is one of the lighter sides of our Alzheimer's stories and I know there are more serious stories coming. I only hope that if and when you suffer or have to care for someone that is suffering from this disease, you can find something that will keep them stimulated. My dad still has the ability to hit the golf ball pretty good and actually shot six under in the qualifying round a couple of weeks ago. The other players that qualified from the same course shot one under and even par. The USGA didn't make an exception for my dad, they simply disqualified him because he could not remember what he shot on a particular hole and therefore could not verify his scores following the round. They rethought their decision and realized that this decision was unfair to golfers that suffered some sort of handicap and my father certainly has a handicap. I think they made the correct decision by reversing their decision. It was not an exception. It was simply the right thing to do. Playing golf is the one thing we've found that stimulates him. Dad's really a great person and if you have any doubts about his qualifications for being here, he should be nailing the 200 yard sign just about now."

Abe had arrived and was sitting in the stands, a little closer to where Charlie was hitting. "Hey Charlie, hit the sign," he yelled.

Almost as if it was on cue, Charlie's next shot was a solid three iron that hit the sign squarely in the middle. "Thwonnnk," went the sign as Mikey smiled at the fans and asked "how many of the golfers here can do that on cue?"

Mikey walked back to where Charlie was setting up to hit the sign again. "Thwonnnk," went the sign as Charlie's ball this time hit in almost the exact same spot.

Mikey turned toward Abe and winked. However, he didn't see the expression of the fans' faces but he could only imagine what they were thinking. "Way to go, Dad. Let's go play some golf," he added.

As Mikey and Charlie walked by the fans that were talking earlier, one of them came up and said, "Good luck Mister Caldwell. You have a great swing, sir and we'll be following you on Thursday."

Charlie smiled and said, "Okay."

Before Charlie and Mikey could turn away, the fan had one last request. "Sir, would you please sign my cap?"

"Okay," replied Charlie as he took the cap and using the felt tip marker, signed a rough-looking "Charlie."

"There you go, fella," Charlie said as he handed the cap back to the fan.

Mikey turned and nodded a thank you to the group of fans still sitting on the bleachers before taking Charlie's hand and leading him to the exit. He and Charlie left the range and went straight to the first tee without going to the putting green.

There were no other golfers even close to being ready to go so Mikey had Charlie tee up a ball. With the exception of having Abe around, they would be by themselves today. "Dad, let's favor the right side of the fairway but we don't want to be in the rough. Okay? Aim this shot toward that tree at the end of the fairway."

"Okay," replied Charlie, as he hit the perfect shot as ordered by Mikey.

This practice round was not so much for Charlie as it was for Mikey. He would be managing the course and simply telling Charlie where to hit certain shots based upon the pin position. As they played each hole, he imagined what would be the best position for Charlie to aim for so that he would have the best chance to make birdie. Charlie's strength was the wedge so Mikey looked at each hole to see what shots would give him the best chance to make birdie.

After eighteen holes, Mikey had a real good idea on where Charlie would have to hit the ball to score and which areas he should avoid. With this information, they were ready.

Abe was right there as they finished. Mikey told Abe that they were done for the day and they were going to take a drive around the city. "I don't know for sure what we'll do but it won't be golf. I'd like to drive up to the lake and see what's up there. Do you want to come along?" Mikey asked.

"No, I'll hang around the golf course and watch some of the golf," Abe said. "I'll be with you guys on Thursday though."

With that, Mikey and Charlie headed back to the hotel and went up to the room. Mikey called home and spoke to his Mom.

"Mom, we've just finished our practice round for today and we're back in the hotel now. Dad wanted to give you a call to see how you're doing."

"Mikey, I'm just fine and was hoping you'd call and let me know how things were going. Have you had any problems with your dad?" she asked.

"Nah, we haven't had any problems at all. Of course, he has problems remembering names of people but occasionally something triggers his memory. Oh yes, guess who showed up yesterday?" Mikey asked.

"I don't have any idea," responded Diane.

"Abe showed up. He flew in from San Antonio yesterday. We had dinner with him last night and asked if he wanted to join us this afternoon. He said that he would rather hang around the course and watch some of the other golf."

"That is fantastic news," replied Diane. "I know that Charlie will appreciate Abe cheering him on."

She paused for a moment. "Mikey, it is good that you're there with Charlie. I think deep down inside he knows you're his son. Hang in there," she added.

"I will, Mom," he added. "Do you want to talk to dad?"

"Sure, let me talk to him."

"Dad, Mom's on the phone and wants to say hi to you," Mikey said as he held the phone out for his father.

Charlie held the phone to his ear and said, "Hi Diane. Are you in… in…?" Charlie momentarily lost the name of the city before coming up with a different way to ask it, "Are you home?"

"Yes Charlie, I'm still in San Antonio. Mikey tells me that you've been playing some really good golf. Do you like the course there?" she asked.

"It's Okay, "he replied. "They got new balls for practicing here. I'm not kidding either. We hit a bucket of balls today that was full of brand new Titleist golf balls."

"That is great, Charlie. You should always have new balls when playing golf," she replied. "You played yesterday and today. Are you going somewhere this afternoon?"

"Mikey says we're going to go to a lake. I can't remember the name but it's a big lake," Charlie said.

"Yes, I think it is Lake Ontario and it is a big lake. It should be very pretty."

"We could go home and pick you up," said Charlie. He turned toward Mikey and asked, "Mikey, can we go and pick up Diane?"

"No, Dad, Mom lives in San Antonio and that is too far away. If we do this again, we'll take her with us," replied Mikey from across the room.

"Mikey says we can't go home to pick you us this time but maybe next time."

"Okay, Charlie. I'll promise to go with you guys next time. I want you to have lots of fun today and enjoy the lake. You should have a good time with Mikey," Diane said.

"Okay," replied Charlie.

Charlie finished the call with Diane and hung up the phone

They had a quick lunch at the hotel and then drove north to the edge of Lake Ontario. "Dad, we can't go north any further. Should we go east or west?" Mikey asked.

"Let's go east," replied Charlie.

Mikey turned the car right and headed east on Lake Shore Drive. After driving for about thirty minutes or so, they came to a beautiful spot on the shores of Lake Ontario called Sodus Point. Stopping at a local museum next to one of the large berthing areas, the two went inside to see some beautifully preserved sailing boats from the Eighteenth and Nineteenth Century. Charlie's interest showed as he was really enjoying looking at some old boats that used to work the lake.

After leaving the museum, they had an early dinner at one of the local diners and then headed back to the hotel. All in all, it was the perfect day for both. Charlie was relaxed and could forget about playing golf while Mikey just enjoyed the time with his dad.

Arriving back at the hotel, Mikey called and got the tee time for tomorrow's round and who they would be playing with. They were paired with Bob Gilder and Dan Morres who was a qualifier from right here in Rochester. The group was going off at 8:30am in the morning.

Chapter Nine

Both, Charlie and Mikey were already up and through most of their morning tasks when the wake-up call came. Charlie picked it up and tried to carry on a conversation with the automated voice message system.

"Mikey, they won't tell me who it is," he said with some anxiety.

"Dad, it's just the wake-up call I put in for last night. I told them to give us a call at 5:45am in the morning. Look at the clock. See, it's 5:45am."

"Okay, but I'm trying to tell you the person on the other end wouldn't say who they were," replied Charlie.

"I don't know who it was but we'll check at the desk," said Mikey without having any plan on checking anything at the desk. He knew his father wouldn't remember the call after a few minutes anyway.

They had a fairly quick breakfast and Charlie again had his favorite, pancakes.

It was time to head to the course and get a little practice in before the 8:30am tee time.

Tee times for Thursday started at 7:30am so the practice range had ten or eleven professionals, all hitting balls with precision. A few of the big names had their coaches, giving comments and last-minute corrections.

Charlie and Mikey entered the area and walked up to an empty space where balls had already been placed. Mikey handed his dad the golf glove that he used yesterday and pulled out the nine-iron as the club he would use to begin his warm up.

Charlie looked at the glove and was trying to put in on the wrong hand. "No, Dad, the glove goes on your left hand, remember?"

"Okay," replied Charlie.

Mikey had to help him with the glove, but soon had it on. He handed Charlie the nine-iron and told him to hit the balls directly over the one hundred hard sign. Charlie didn't have to think on this and hit each ball precisely over the sign. There was soon a small circle of balls lying near each other about one hundred and twenty yards from the tee.

The same practice and results were achieved with the other irons and then came the woods. When Mikey handed him the driver, Charlie looked at it and said, "I like the driver, Mikey. It goes far."

"That's right, Dad. The driver goes far. Aim at the two-fifty sign and see if you can get it there in the air."

"Okay," replied Charlie.

He hit several drivers and Mikey watched intently. The driver was the one club in the bag that varied on distance. Charlie would hit a ball that carried two hundred and sixty yards and the very next one would only go two hundred and twenty yards. The swing would be the same, the balls are identical and Mikey thought it could be the driver. However, trying to get Charlie to change would almost be impossible.

Mikey glanced at the clock on the practice range and saw that there was 45 minutes before they were to tee off. "Dad, we got about 45 minutes before we play golf so let's go putt a few balls on the practice green."

"Okay," replied Charlie.

Charlie putted balls from various lengths and was pretty accurate with most. He had a slight problem with distance as the green was much faster today than it had been earlier in the week. Never the less, he was always right around the hole when he missed.

It was now time to make their way to the tee box and the two walked over through the crowd. Bob Gilder and Dan Morres were the other two players in the group and both were already on the tee box.

Dan walked over and introduced himself, "Hello, I'm Dan Morres."

Charlie shook Dan's hand and said, "Hi, I'm Charlie. Are you playing golf with me today?"

Dan knew that the third player had Alzheimer's and was somewhat prepared. He simply answered, "Yes, Charlie, we're playing golf together. Let's have some fun."

"Okay," replied Charlie.

Bob Gilder walked over as Charlie and Dan were talking and made the first introduction. "Hello Charlie. My name is Bob Gilder and it is my pleasure to being playing golf with you today."

"Hi, Bob, my name is Charlie."

Bob smiled at Charlie and added, "Charlie, my dad had Alzheimer's. He used to play golf but I never asked him to play after we found out he had it. I wish I would have taken him out to the course now."

"Oh, that's too bad," said Charlie. "Tell you what, ask your dad if he wants to play today," Charlie added.

"Oh, my dad is not here, Charlie. He's gone now."

"That is too bad, we could have had fun if he was here," Charlie added.

It was now time as the group in front had cleared the fairway. The announcer held the microphone and announced, "Group Number six with a tee time of eight-thirty. From right here in Rochester, welcome Dan Morres." Dan acknowledged the small crowd as he was clearly the favorite in the group, walked up to the tee and teed his ball. He took several practice swings that were very smooth. He stepped up to the ball and the swing was not like his practice swings. It was much faster and the ball headed down the fairway and was slicing into the edge of the woods on the right.

Charlie watched Dan's ball and said, "It looked like that one went right."

"First tee jitters," replied Dan very quietly.

The announcer now said, "From San Antonio, Texas, welcome Charlie Caldwell. The crowd clapped politely as Charlie stood there."

"Dad, it's your turn to hit," Mikey said. "Put this right down the middle."

"Okay," replied Charlie, as he walked up and put his used Titleist golf ball on the tee. He stood behind the ball for a second then took the one practice swing, stepped up and took the same swing as the practice. The ball took off straight down the middle of the fairway, landing just short of the area where the fairway slopes toward the green. The ball hit the slope and bounded down another 30 yards, stopping in the center of the fairway, about 140 yards from the green.

The crowd clapped loudly and Mikey heard someone say, "That's the best one so far."

"Nice shot, Dad," Mikey said.

"Nice shot," Bob said, as he began walking to the tee.

The announcer said, "From Corvalis, Oregon, welcome Bob Gilder." Again, the crowd clapped.

After teeing his ball, Bob stood behind his ball and concentrated on the fairway. "Follow Charlie's ball," he said as he walked up and addressed his shot. His ball took the same flight as Charlie's, but had a slight draw and it ended up in the short rough at about the same distance.

The forecaddies had already found Dan's shot and he was blocked from moving forward. He had to chip back to the fairway and had over two hundred and twenty yards to the green. His third shot again went right into the woods.

Bob was slightly farther away than Charlie so he hit first. It was a great shot that rose high and landed on the green, stopping immediately. He had a twenty foot putt for birdie.

Mikey looked at the pin placement sheet and his notes and picked the landing spot for Charlie's ball. He handed his dad an eight-iron and said, "Dad, here's your club. Hit it just over the sand trap and the ball should turn toward the hole."

"Okay," replied Charlie.

Charlie took the eight-iron and addressed the ball. He took the one practice swing and then hit the shot that Mikey asked for. The ball landed about ten feet past the bunker, took a short hop and began rolling toward the hole. It stopped about five feet below the hole.

Dan scrambled around in the woods and ended up carding an eight on the first hole and was basically out of the tournament at that point. He was nervous and the first hole took whatever golf game he had and destroyed it. He would end up shooting an eighty-nine to put him out of the tournament.

Bob Gilder missed his birdie and Charlie made his.

"Nice birdie," said Bob as Charlie reached down to retrieve his ball from the hole.

Mikey placed the flag back and added, "Nice putt, Dad."

"Okay," replied Charlie.

The second hole was a bit tighter than the first, but it was some fifty yards shorter. Bob and Charlie both hit respectable drives and Charlie was first to hit the second shot.

Mikey looked at the pin placement sheet and looked at his notes for the second hole. "Dad, we don't want to be long on this one so let's go for the center of the green." He was about one hundred and twenty yards so Mikey handed him a nine-iron.

Charlie hit the shot that Mikey asked for. It hit in the center of the green, then began spinning backwards. The ball hit a severe down slope and backed all the way off the green.

"That ball rolled back off the green," Charlie said.

"Yes, you just hit it too good, Dad. It hit up on top but the spin pulled it back down. We should be able to get up and down though," Mikey said.

Bob Gilder saw what happened to Charlie's ball and he changed his target to a bit higher on the green. His shot flew high and true, landing and stopping about five feet from the cup.

Charlie chipped up and made his par while Bob made his birdie.

Both players matched pars on the next few holes and were both one under when they came to the relatively short par-three Number Six. Mikey measured the distance from the tee to the pin at 167 yards and realized a full six iron would be perfect.

Bob was still hitting first and thought long and hard about club selection, finally picking a seven iron. Mikey glanced at Bob's bag and realized he was hitting a seven iron. He watched intently as Bob's ball flew toward the pin but hit a few yards short of the green and bounced backwards. This left him with a very difficult chip up the steep hill.

Mikey handed Charlie a six iron and gave him instructions to go directly at the flag. Charlie repeated his tee shot routine and hit a low-flying ball that was heading directly at the pin. The ball hit a few feet short of the pin, took a bounce and hit the pin solidly. It dropped straight down, ending up just inches from the hole.

"Great shot, Dad," exclaimed Mikey. "I thought it was going to be short at first then was worried it was going to bounce over the back. Even if it missed the flag, it wouldn't have gone far. That was fantastic, Dad."

Bob Gilder chipped up and missed the six foot putt, leaving him at even par after six. Charlie made the tap in and was at two under for the round.

Both players made par on holes seven through nine and Charlie was two under at the turn, while Bob Gilder was even par.

Mikey looked at the scoreboard near the eighteenth green as they walked to the number ten tee box. "Look, Dad, you're leading the tournament at two under par."

"Okay," replied Charlie.

Charlie pushed his tee shot on number ten and it was one of those drives that didn't go very far. It was a few feet in the rough, while Bob Gilder boomed a drive and had around one hundred yards to the pin. Mikey surveyed Charlie's position and determined that the best shot would be to hit a medium iron to the fairway and leave a short wedge or sand wedge to the green. He thought there would be too much risk to try and reach the green that was about 190 yards away. He handed Charlie a six iron and said, "Dad, let's go for just in front of the green. That will leave a short pitch shot and that's your favorite shot."

Charlie looked at the club and addressed the ball. He stopped his routine and turned back to Mikey. "Mikey, I don't think I can reach the green with this club."

"I know Dad. I think it would be best to hit short of the green, and then chip up for your par."

"No! I don't want to lay up. You see where that fella's ball is? He's way down there and I'm way back here. I need something that will reach the green," Charlie added.

"Okay, Dad, here's a five-wood for you to hit. That will get you to the green. If you miss it, you could be in big trouble," Mikey said as he handed the five-wood to his dad and took the six-iron back. "Aim for the middle of the green," he added.

Charlie addressed the ball with the five-wood and took his usual, routine practice swing. He then took the same swing and hit a low shot that never climbed higher than a few feet off the ground. It was heading left of the hole but was turning right. It hit short of the green and bounced just right of the large bunker protecting the front. It rolled up the green and stopped twenty feet from the pin.

Charlie looked at Mikey and said, "That was fun."

"Great shot, Dad! I was worried but you pulled it off."

Up ahead, Bob watched the shot and thought the best thing would be to do what Mikey suggested. When he saw Charlie swinging the fairway wood, he thought to himself that this ball could go anywhere. He never expected it to even come close to the green, let alone end up just twenty feet from the pin.

After he watched Charlie's shot, Bob went to his bag and grabbed his wedge. "We've got to get this close," he said to his caddie.

Bob's wedge flew directly over the flag and spun back to just inches away from the cup. It looked like it was going in but stopped at the last moment. "I thought we'd made it," he said to his caddie as he changed clubs to his putter.

Charlie took a quick glance at the line and looked back to Mikey. He was asking for instructions on the break but it was not verbal. Mikey looked at the break again from both sides and said, "Dad, this looks like the putt will break to the left but I think it is actually straight. Let's go straight at the hole"

"Okay," replied Charlie.

Charlie stepped up to the ball and took the usual one practice stroke. He then struck the ball sending it on a line straight at the hole. It ran straight and true, dropping into the center of the cup.

Charlie smiled and looked back at Mikey. "Nice putt, huh?"

"Yeah, Dad, that was a pretty nice putt."

"Nice birdie," said Bob Gilder.

Charlie was now three under par and Bob Gilder was one under as they came up to the extremely difficult par three, number eleven. It was a narrow fairway with a long and narrow green. The pin was placed in the back, leaving two hundred and twelve yards to the pin.

Crowds were watching the leader board and noticed that the new golfer, Charlie Caldwell, was on number eleven, and he was leading the tournament at three under. More and more fans began to follow this group.

As Charlie was walking up to the tee, one of the fans said out loud, "hit the pin, Charlie."

Charlie didn't look to see who said this but simply replied, "Okay."

Mikey did look at the person who said this and it was the same one that he talked with early Tuesday morning. Mikey acknowledged the fan and said, "Hi, how are you doing today?"

"We're doing really well and we're glad Charlie is doing well. Keep it up."

"Thanks, he's trying and giving everything he's got," Mikey replied as he turned back to Charlie.

"Dad, we're over two hundred yards to this pin. I think we should go for it. What do you think?"

"Okay," replied Charlie.

Mikey handed Charlie the beat-up five-wood that literally looked like it just came from a second-hand store. It was an old wooden club and the varnish was peeling off. Charlie teed a ball then took the usual practice swing. What followed was what Bob Gilder would later say that day was the very best golf shot he's ever witnessed.

Charlie hit the five-wood on the screws and it started off to the right side of the green and turned ever so slightly to the left. It landed on the right front of the green and began rolling to the right of the hole. As it ran up, it began turning toward the hole. It looked like it was going in and the fans around the green were making loud expressions.

Bob Gilder watched it and said, "It's going in Charlie."

Charlie watched and saw the ball spin around the hole and the gasp from the audience confirmed he barely missed the shot. It actually spun completely around the hole and ended up six inches away.

The crowd around the tee box was now extremely loud and the fan from Tuesday started a chant. "Charlie… Charlie… "Most of the fans surrounding the tee box picked up on the chant and soon everyone was repeating it.

After the crowd quieted down, Bob Gilder walked up to the tee box and hit a three-iron that went right and stayed right all the way. He had a difficult chip and ended up with a bogey on the hole.

Charlie made his tap in to go four under for the day and the chants of "Charlie… Charlie…" got louder and louder as the day progressed.

Putting for a basic par on the last hole, Charlie ended his round with a four under sixty-seven. Bob Gilder had an even par seventy-one and Dan Morres had an eighty-nine.

The golfers all shook hands and Bob Gilder and Dan Morres both commented on Charlie's excellent round. "Very nice round, Charlie," said Dan Morres.

"Okay," replied Charlie.

As they walked off the green, Charlie heard Abe call out. "There's the All or Nothing Guy, great round, Charlie."

Charlie looked up and made eye contact with Abe. "Hey there," he said back. "It was a good round, wasn't it? What did I end up with?"

Charlie didn't wait for Abe to say anything or answer the question. He simply turned away and looked around for Mikey. Mikey saw Abe and told him they'd see him after they recorded the scores.

Mikey went into the scoring booth with Charlie and reviewed the score card that had been filled out by Dan Morres. Mikey verified the card matched the one he kept for Charlie. Once he verified all the scores, he handed it to Charlie and showed him where to sign.

"Here you go, Dad," he said as he handed the score card to his Dad and watched him sign the card. "Nice round."

"Did I make par?" Charlie asked?

"You were actually four under par, Dad. Lots of other golfers are still on the course but you are the current leader."

"Sixty-seven! That's a really great round, Charlie," said Bob Gilder as he handed his signed card to the official behind the desk. "I played my ass off and was lucky to be even par. Some of these greens are like trying to stop a marble on top of a watermelon."

"Watermelon," said Charlie. "I like watermelon."

Charlie signed his card with a simple "Charlie" and handed it to the official. The official checked the card and re-added the numbers. "Sixty-seven, Mister Caldwell that is a very good round."

"Okay," replied Charlie.

"Let's go to the locker room," Mikey said.

Immediately after leaving the scoring trailer, Charlie and Mikey were surrounded by fans and news media wanting an interviewer. ESPN had preference on location and was the first to grab Charlie. "Mister Caldwell," the ESPN reported called out. "Can we have a few words with you?" he asked.

Mikey stepped in front of his father. "Sir, my dad will grant an interview but I need to be there with him. Can we go to another location?" he asked.

"Sure," replied the ESPN announcer. "We can go to the club house. We have a room setup for interviews."

They walked into the club house and we ushered into a small room that resembled a library area. Lights were already on and they had Charlie sit in one of the chairs in front of a large bank of lights.

After the ESPN reporter sat down and the camera crew reported that they were ready, the announcer began. "Mister Caldwell," he said, "That was a super round you had. We had you missing only one fairway and you hit fourteen out of eighteen greens in regulation. How would you describe your round?"

Charlie looked at the announcer, then at the camera. He paused for a second or two and then said, "It was Okay," he replied.

The announcer then said, "The fairway wood you hit on the par three on the back side was the best of the day. Let's review this so you can tell the folks what you thought when the ball left the club."

They rolled the tape and Charlie watched the shot on the monitor. "That was a good golf shot," he said.

"Did you think it was going in the hole?" the announcer asked.

"I don't remember what I thought, but look at the television here. It almost went in, huh?"

"Yes," replied the announcer. "I see that your son is also your caddie. Can we ask him a couple of questions?"

"Yes, Mikey is my caddie," replied Charlie.

"Mikey, the story about you and your father is amazing and is one of the most popular golf stories we've had in several years. Do you find that your father is handicapped in any way?"

"Well, things are not always easy out there. Dad has a strange disease and it has created lots of issues for sure. Dad often forgets where he's at and what he did on the last shot. I look at the situation and decide where our target should be. I then pick out the club for him and tell him where to hit it. Dad then takes over and applies some amazing physical skills to put the ball where I told him to hit it," Mikey said smiling.

"Mikey, let's go over what you both did on number eleven today. That was a remarkable shot and it almost went in. How did you go about telling your dad which club to hit and where to aim the shot?" the announcer asked.

"Well, we just came off a fantastic birdie on ten. I wanted dad to lay up but he said he could reach the green. I really tried to talk him out of it but he had his 'All or Nothing' attitude and I knew I would not be able to get him to play the safe shot. I gave him a five-wood and he played a low cut that rolled right up to the pin. Personally, I think that shot was better than the one on the par three. On the par three, I handed dad the same five-wood and told him to aim at the center of the green. He normally hits a pretty straight ball so when this began heading for the right side of the green, I was afraid we'd miss it right. He had a bit of a draw and the ball turned back toward the center of the green. It hit, bounced forward and kept turning toward the hole. We couldn't see it but we learned later that it lipped out on the right side of the cup."

122

"What are you going to do to get ready for tomorrow's round," the announcer asked.

"Well, dad heard Bob Gilder describe the greens as being difficult to keep the ball on them and I think he said it was like trying to balance a marble on top of a watermelon. Dad heard the watermelon part of the story so we're going to go get a cold watermelon. We will stop by a park on the way back to the hotel and eat a cold watermelon. That's what we'll do to prepare for tomorrow."

They tried to ask some more questions but Mikey refused to take any more questions and took Charlie to the locker room to change his shoes. They then headed to the car. Abe was waiting for them when they exited the club house and they talked about when they'd be playing on Friday.

"I checked the board and you're off at One-thirty tomorrow afternoon," said Abe.

"Yeah, that's what I saw earlier. We're heading back to the hotel now and stopping on the way to get a watermelon. Care to join us?" asked Mikey.

"No, I'm going to try to catch Watson and Player. They just went off the first tee and I'll catch them on the second or third hole. It's not very often that you can see this level of golf talent. I'll catch you both tomorrow. Get lots of rest," Abe added.

Mikey and Charlie left the Oak Hill Country Club and stopped by a large super market. They walked in and went straight to the produce section. Charlie remembered something about tapping the watermelon to see if it was fresh and he tapped a large one in the bin. "Thummmp" was the echoing cry from the melon as it responded to Charlie's finger.

"Mikey, this one sounds real good. Let's get this one," Charlie said with the excitement of a ten year old.

Mikey lifted the watermelon and the two walked to the registers. Mikey paid for the melon and the two were soon in the park. They had to borrow a plastic knife to cut the melon but soon were sitting on a park bench in Rochester, New York, eating sweet, cold watermelon.

Mikey enjoyed the moment with his father. It was just the two of them, sitting in a park and eating watermelon. The only thing missing that would have capped the day off as being perfect would be having the ability to go over the first round of the US Senior Open, shot by shot. This was something that Charlie could not do.

When they arrived back to the DoubleTree, they turned on the television and watched the rest of the field finishing up on day one. One by one, new scores were posted and four under was still leading the pack. Day one's official final had Charlie leading at four under and Jay Hass, Bernard Langer and Tom Watson were all tied with Bob Gilder at even par.

Chapter Ten

Mikey was sleeping very soundly and it was like he was in a dream. It sounded as if someone was banging on a wall or slamming a door shut. "Stop slamming that damn door," he thought. But the noise of the door slamming against the frame and the loud sound of the bells hanging from the door knob kept getting louder and louder and eventually caused him to wake up and set up in bed.

"Dad," he said quite loudly. What are you doing up and why are you banging on the door?

"I want to go see Diane," Charlie replied. "I need to see Diane. She needs me and I want to go home now."

Mikey glanced at the clock on the night stand. "Dad, it's three-thirty in the morning. You need to get some rest."

Charlie was still looking at the door and trying to get it open. Crying this time, he called out, "Diane...Diane, come and get me. They won't let me out."

Mikey quickly got out of bed and walked over to where his dad was trying to open the door. "Dad, we will see Diane in a couple of days. Remember, we called her on the telephone yesterday. She was just fine and she wanted you to have a good time. Don't you remember talking with her yesterday?"

"I don't remember talking with Diane. Where is she?" Charlie cried out.

"Dad... Dad," Mikey called out trying to reassure his father. "Mom is in San Antonio and we're in New York. We will be flying back to San Antonio in three more days. Here, let's go back to bed and get some rest. We've got a busy day tomorrow."

"I want to see Diane," Charlie kept crying out. "I want to see Diane."

"Dad, just relax for a moment. I'll get something that will help you," he said as he turned and walked into the bathroom.

Mikey found what he was looking for and returned with a small spray bottle. He read the instructions again. It read, Paroxetine – Spray one full spray under the tongue or toward the back of the mouth. Do not exceed one spray every two hours. "Here, Dad, open your mouth. This will make you feel better."

Surprisingly, Charlie opened his mouth and Mikey sprayed the solution toward the base of the tongue.

Charlie coughed and gagged a bit. "That shit is no good, Mikey."

"It will help you relax, Dad. Here, drink this water too. It will help get rid of the taste?"

"Okay," replied Charlie.

Mikey gave his dad a glass of water and within minutes the Paroxetine was beginning to work. Charlie had calmed down and Mikey talked him into lying down for a few minutes. It worked and Charlie was soon fast asleep.

It took Mikey a while longer to go back to sleep as he kept wondering if what he was doing for his father was the best thing. After all, Charlie didn't realize that he was actually playing in the US Senior Open. He was just thinking he was playing a friendly game of golf in front of a lot of people. Was it the best thing for his father?

After a fitful night's sleep, Mikey woke up. He looked at the clock and it was seven-thirty. Charlie was still asleep, lying on his back, snoring slightly.

Mikey took a hot shower and after drying off, he woke his father. "Dad, it's time to get up," he said, touching his father's shoulder.

Charlie opened his eyes and for a quick moment recognized Mikey as his son. "Good morning, Mikey. What time is it?"

"It's almost eight in the morning. We have plenty of time so there's no hurry. Why don't you take a hot shower and I'll figure out what we'll wear today."

"Okay," replied Charlie as he turned and got out of bed.

They had a leisurely breakfast and even called Diane before heading to the course at eleven thirty.

Unlike the previous days, an entourage of reporters and fans surrounded Charlie and Mikey as they walked from their car to the entrance of the club house. Fans were lined up for autographs and it was fortunate that Mikey talked with his father about signing autographs. He told him that there would be lots of people that would come up and ask him for his autograph. Mikey told him to use the black marker and just sign 'Charlie.'

Fans handed Charlie hats, shirts, programs, and a sundry of other items. Charlie became quite adept at signing his name real quick and handing it back to the person. Some fans would ask for the signature to be to a person and Charlie would simply say, "Okay," but still sign it just Charlie.

The press and the cameras were eating this up and there were dozens of camera crews trying to get the perfect shot of the professional golfer with Alzheimer's. Some even asked questions like, "Charlie, how do you like playing in the Senior Open?" Charlie was always polite, but usually just said, "Okay."

After signing hundreds of autographs, the two finally made it to the sanctuary of the club house. Fans or members of the press were not allowed in the club house and therefore, there were no autograph seekers. Occasionally, one of the other professional golfers would ask Charlie to autograph a glove or ball and usually said it was a request from a family member. Fred Couples was in the locker when Mikey and Charlie walked in and Fred walked up to Mikey and said, "I'm really sorry to bother you in the locker room, but could you ask your dad to sign this glove. It's for my mother and she specifically asked if I could get Charlie to sign this glove."

"Sure," he said as he took the glove and handed it to Charlie. "Here, Dad, will you sign this glove for Fred Couples."

Charlie took the glove and signed it with 'Charlie.' He handed it back to Fred and asked, "Are you Fred?"

Fred Couples was not accustomed to people asking him if he was Fred and smiled with a huge grin. "Yes, I am Fred Couples. It is a pleasure to meet you Charlie."

"You look like a golfer. Are you going to play golf today?" Charlie asked.

"I play golf and one of these days, I'd love to play a round with you, Charlie."

"Okay," replied Charlie.

128

After Fred left, Charlie sat down and put on his golf shoes. "That was a nice guy. I wish he would play golf with us." Like many conversations Charlie made lately, he would completely change direction in the middle. Such was the case here, when he paused a second before asking, "Why does everyone want me to sign my name, Mikey?"

"I don't know," replied Mikey. "I guess it's just because you're a special person and they love watching you play golf. I like watching you play golf too."

"Okay, we'll play golf today," replied Charlie.

As they left the sanctuary of the club house and headed for the practice area, Charlie was again hounded for autographs. He gladly began signing everything handed to him. Mikey had to intervene and drag Charlie through the crowd as fast as possible. A couple of security people saw the problem and that the fans were keeping Charlie and Mikey penned in so they made an opening.

Soon, they were through the crowd and on the practice tee. There were a couple of free areas in the middle of the areas so Mikey led Charlie there. He set the clubs down and got a bucket of new Titleist golf balls, putting them down next to where Charlie would begin his warm-up routine.

"Look, Mikey, they got new golf balls and they're all Titleist!" he said as he took a ball from the bucket and examined it. "We should take a bunch of these balls home."

"We can't take the balls home, Dad. They're for practice only," replied Mikey as he handed his dad a pitching wedge to begin the routine. "Here, hit some balls and let's see if you can hit the hundred yard sign."

"Okay," replied Charlie.

He dropped the ball he was holding and used the wedge to move it to a good piece of grass. Charlie took a smooth practice swing then used the same swing again, hitting the ball on a line directly at the one hundred yard sign. It hit the small, circular sign directly in the middle and it gave off a fairly loud "thwoonnnk."

Charlie and Mikey both heard the comments from the fans that were standing in the area behind the golfers. Many fans clapped when the ball hit the sign.

The second ball looked like it was also going to hit the sign but missed by inches. As it missed, the crowd could be heard building up to a crescendo but ending in an "Auhhhhhhhh."

The third shot again looked like it was heading straight for the sign. When it hit, Mikey barely heard the "thwoonnnk" before the sound was drowned out by the clapping from the crowd. As their clapping quieted down, Charlie turned and smiled at his new fans. It was very obvious that he was beginning to really enjoy this.

Mikey noticed this change in his father's attitude and said softly, "Dad, give the crowd a small hand jester, kind of like you're giving a small wave to them. They will love it."

"You want me to wave at the crowd?" he asked.

"Yes, Dad, wave at the crowd when they clap," responded Mikey.

"Okay," replied Charlie as he got another ball ready to hit. Again, the ball flew straight at the sign, hitting it for two times in a row. This time the crowd really erupted in a loud applause, which Charlie acknowledged with a small wave of the hand.

Mikey looked down the line of other golfers warming up and saw that several had stopped and were also watching Charlie. "Okay Dad, let's hit it one more time," said Mikey quietly to his father.

Charlie again used the wedge to free up one new Titleist and moved it to a new spot in the closely cut grass. Again the short practice swing, followed by the same real one. The ball was a bit higher in flight this time but still managed to come down in time to hit the sign for three times in a row. This time, not only the crowd clapped enthusiastically, but they were joined by many of the other golf pros. Again, Charlie just simply raised his hand in a small wave like a celebrity in a parade.

Charlie could continue to hit wedges as long as the crowd enjoyed it but Mikey had the nine-iron for him to hit next. "Let's hit these directly over the one hundred yard sign."

"Okay," replied Charlie.

Like with the wedge, ball after ball took the same flight path as the others. It was similar results with the other clubs too. Mikey didn't want to cause any additional disturbance so he instructed Charlie to aim away from the signs, which Charlie did.

After slowly working their way through each club in Charlie's bag, Mikey checked the clock near the practice range. It was now about thirty minutes before their tee time and they followed Bob Gilder as he left the practice area and headed for the practice green.

Bob slowed down a bit so Charlie could catch up. As Charlie came even, Bob said "Let's have another sixty-seven, Charlie."

"Okay," replied Charlie.

He didn't recognize Bob Gilder and later asked Mikey, "Who was that guy that walked over here with us?"

"That's Bob Gilder, Dad. He's a professional golfer and he will be playing with us today."

"Okay," replied Charlie.

Placing three balls on the practice green, Charlie took the old Arnold Palmer blade putter and was showing great form. Ball after ball rolled directly in the hole from three feet, five feet and eight feet. When he made two in a row from over fifteen feet, Mikey could hear the crowd behind talking. Though he wasn't able to distinguish individual conversations, he knew they were very impressed with his dad's putting skills.

After what seemed to be an eternity, the group was finally called to the tee and the group walked through the crowd and on to the teeing area. The announcer made the call. "Ladies and gentlemen, from San Antonio, Texas, with an opening round of sixty-seven, please welcome Charlie Caldwell."

Charlie placed a ball on a tee and looked down the tee box to the fairway. As far as he could see, people lined both sides of the hole. He stepped back and looked at Mikey. "Mikey, these people are too close. If I miss the ball, it could hit one of them."

Mikey walked over and whispered in Charlie's ear, "Dad, they're here to watch you hit it down the middle. Aim for the middle of the fairway and forget that the people are here."

"Okay," replied Charlie.

Stepping back to the ball, Charlie looked up at the people several times and took several practice swings. The practice swings were jerky as was the actual swing hitting the ball. It came off low on the club face and was slicing right. It sliced over the crowd lining the tee box, barely missing a few of the fans.

There was silence from the crowd but Charlie again made the small hand wave.

"Ladies and gentlemen, welcome Bob Gilder from Corvallis, Oregon." Bob waved at the crowd and immediately teed a ball and hit it straight down the middle of the fairway. Dan Morres' drive mirrored Bob's and the two of them walked down the path and then down the center of the fairway.

Mikey and Charlie headed down the same path but turned sharply to the right. In the distance Mikey could see the crowd maneuvering for position around Charlie's tee shot. Each person wanted to be as close to the ball as possible.

Mikey noticed his dad was very quiet and said, "Dad, those people were too close. We'll make sure they're not that close to you again."

Charlie simply replied, "Okay."

When they arrived to where Charlie's ball was lying in the thick grass, an official had to move the crowd back. Not satisfied with how far they moved away from the ball, he again ordered them to move further. Charlie felt like he was being smothered by all the people. "Mikey, these people are too close."

"I know. I'll get the officials to move them back." It took several minutes but eventually the officials had everybody moved back enough that Charlie could have a free swing at the ball. Mikey had not planned for hitting a shot from this area and determined that an eight-iron should get them back in the fairway.

Handing his dad an eight-iron, he pointed out where they should land the ball. "Just take a smooth swing, Dad," he said.

Charlie again took several practice swings and again the real swing was not as smooth as usual. He topped the ball and it rolled some about thirty feet before again stopping in the thick grass.

The crowd was talking loud now and Mikey heard several people say things like, "I knew he would choke today." Another one said, "What did I tell you? I knew a person suffering from Alzheimer's couldn't maintain concentration."

"He's done," replied another.

Mikey knew he had to do something quick to turn Charlie around. "What can I do?" he thought to himself.

That was about the time that Abe moved his way through the crowd and was standing a few feet away from Charlie. "Charlie!" he called out fairly loud. "Show me what 'All or Nothing' looks like."

Hearing Abe, Charlie turned as said, "Hey, Abe. How are you? I thought you were in San Antonio."

"I'm fine Charlie. I just came up to watch you win this tournament. It looks like you got yourself into a spot where even the best golfer in the world would have a hard time. Bet you a beer you can't make a double-bogey from here."

"Okay, a beer it is," Charlie replied. "Mikey, hand me a wedge."

Mikey noticed the sudden change in his father. Something was said that caused something in his broken brain to send electrical signals from the memory banks to the cognitive area.

For a brief moment, the original Charlie Caldwell without Alzheimer's was present and this amazed Mikey. "Okay, Dad," he said as he handed his father the wedge.

"Thanks, son," Charlie replied.

He took the one smooth practice swing and followed it with the same swing that flew the ball to the center of the fairway, just short of the two shots from Bob Gilder and Dan Morres.

"Double-up for a bogey, Abe?" Charlie asked Abe.

"You're on," replied Abe.

Abe walked with Charlie and Mikey for a short while, but had to stop when they reached the ropes separating the golfers from the fans. Mikey tried to get Abe on the other side of the ropes but the officials said that would be a violation and couldn't be done. Abe knew this and had already moved away on the outside of the ropes. "That's alright, Charlie, I'll be following you all day. Play well," he said.

Charlie reached his ball and looked around for Abe. He looked at the fans on each side of the fairway but couldn't find the familiar face. "Mikey, where's the guy that was with us a few minutes ago?"

"That was Abe and he can't be inside the ropes, Dad. He's still betting a beer that you won't make a double-bogey."

"Okay," replied Charlie, as he reached out for Mikey to hand him a club.

"Hold on a second while I look at what we have," Mikey said as he looked at the pin placement sheet and his notes. "Okay, we're one hundred and seventy-five yards from the pin. How about a solid and smooth six-iron," he said, passing the club to his father.

As Charlie was addressing the ball, Mikey added, "Make it like it is 'All or Nothing'."

"Okay," replied Charlie.

Mikey noticed that the current Charlie was back now and this one had Alzheimer's.

He took one practice swing and then used his normal, smooth swing to send the ball directly at the flag. The ball hit short of the flag and bounced hard hitting the flag stick. It ended up a good thirty feet to the right of the pin.

Bob Gilder and Dan Morres both hit respectable shots and each had makeable birdie putts. Charlie had a breaking putt over thirty feet just to save a bogey. He lined the putt up, took one practice swing and then putted the ball. It started out well right of the cup and broke to the left as gravity controlled the shot. The ball narrowly missed the cup, ending up just a few inches beyond the hole.

Charlie walked up to the ball and casually tapped the ball in but it completely missed the hole and ended up fifteen feet away.

Mikey couldn't believe what was happening and maybe everyone was right. Charlie may not be able to hold concentration long enough to play a complete tournament. He watched his dad quickly walk to the ball and casually strike it again toward the hole. He missed again but did make the tap in this time. For the first time, Mikey though he may have made the wrong decision by entering his father in the tournament in the first place.

Charlie picked the ball up out of the hole and walked over to where Mikey was standing. Neither person said anything as they watched both, Bob Gilder and Dan Morres make birdie.

It was a short walk over to the tee box for number two. "Charlie, I have you for an eight? Is that correct?" asked Bob.

Charlie looked puzzled and after trying to remember what he shot, he said, "I can't remember. Mikey, did I make par on the last hole?"

"No, Dad, you scored an eight," replied Mikey.

"Okay," replied Charlie.

Mikey turned to Bob and said, "Yes, he scored an eight. He was four on and then four-putted."

Bob could see the discouragement in Mikey's face. "Get him back to playing good golf, Mikey."

"I don't know, Bob. I may have made the wrong decision by entering him in this tournament. There's too much pressure," Mikey said.

"Mikey, that's bullshit. The pressure is all on you, not Charlie. He doesn't understand pressure and any pressure he may have will come from you. Just give him the right club and tell him where to hit it. You do not need to tell him to hit it like it is all or nothing. The term smooth probably confuses him. Telling him where to hit it worked yesterday and it will work today. Don't expect him to respond to anything else you do or say."

Mikey looked at Bob with sincere appreciation, "Thank you Bob. I really appreciate it."

"No problem," replied Bob. "Now let's play some golf."

When it was Charlie's turn to hit the shot on number two, he reached out for Mikey to hand him a club. Mikey had the driver in his hand already and handed to his father. "Dad, hit it directly down the middle. Your target line is the sand trap in front of the green."

"Okay," replied Charlie.

Charlie's ball went exactly where Mikey requested. Mikey measured the next shot at one hundred and thirty-five yards and handed his dad a nine-iron. "Dad, hit this solid and …," he stopped in the middle of the sentence realizing he was passing unnecessary instruction. Changing his choice of words, he said, "Dad, hit this ball over the right side of the bunker. Do you see the bunker?"

"Okay, I see the bunker," he said before hitting the shot Mikey requested.

The ball flew high and straight, landing just past the flag. It took one short bounce and rolled toward the cup. It stopped just inches from the hole. Bob Gilder's putt for birdie came up a bit short and he tapped in for a par. He was standing near the hole when Charlie made his tap-in. "Nice birdie, Charlie," he said.

Charlie made par on the next eight holes and was three over par for the day and one under for the tournament. Mikey looked at the scoreboard when they walked from the ninth green to the tenth tee box. He saw about ten golfers or so that were at two under or better.

"You're playing some great golf Dad. Let's have some fun. This is number eleven and you were really good with your shot yesterday. Let's do the same thing," said Mikey.

"Okay," replied Charlie.

Almost immediately, Mikey realized he had messed up by giving his dad too much information again. He watched him take a couple of practice swings and suddenly stopped him. "Hold the swing, Dad," he yelled out.

Charlie looked a bit surprised and stepped away from the ball.

Mikey walked up and said, "Dad, hit this one on the right side of the green."

"Okay," replied Charlie.

Charlie addressed the ball with the beat up five-wood and took a beautiful practice swing. The actual swing with the ball was an exact duplicate of the practice swing. The ball took off on a straight line toward the right side of the green. It climbed to about seventy-five feet and was heading toward the requested target. It landed midway between the front and back of the green and stopped.

Mikey had hoped for similar bounce to yesterday's ball on the same hole but the greens were softer today. As a result, Charlie would have a fifty-foot putt that broke left and then hard right at the end.

Mikey studied the putt and picked out a starting line that was aimed about four feet left of the hole. He pointed at the aiming point and said, "This is your target line."

Charlie lined the putt up and sent the ball running toward the spot in the grass that Mikey pointed to. At first the ball turned a bit left and began a climb up a ridge on the green before hitting the severe downslope with a strong right turn. The ball looked as if it wasn't going to make it to the top but barely inched up to the crest before stopping.

"Oh no," said Mikey softly as he realized the next putt would be unbelievably difficult. He realized that it would be impossible to stop the ball from rolling at least several feet past the cup.

Charlie watched the ball and looked surprised when it stopped. He looked at Mikey and had a questioning frown with his eyebrows crunched down. Charlie looked back to the green and took one step toward the ball when he noticed the most miniscule movement with the ball. Charlie stopped in his tracks and watched. To his and everyone else's surprise, the ball ever so slightly turned and began rolling toward the cup. Picking up speed with each inch of the tightly-mowed green, the ball hit the center of the cup and went straight up in the air. As it dropped back down into the cup, the applause from the gallery was deafening. The applause quickly turned into a couple of thousand people in unison shouting, "Charlie... Charlie."

Charlie smiled and did his parade wave.

Bob Gilder was next to putt and walked up as Charlie was retrieving the ball from the cup. Bob stuck out his fist to Charlie for a fist-tap. "Charlie, I think your fans are back in force," he said as the two golfers tapped their fists together lightly.

Charlie made par on the remaining holes of the round and ended up with a two over for the day and two under for the tournament. Bernard Langer played earlier in the day and was leading the tournament as six under. He was followed by Tom Watson who, as usual, was always the crowd favorite at five under.

As authorized by the USGA, Mikey went into the scoring tent with his father. He quickly verified Dan Morres' scores and then passed the card to Charlie, showing him where to sign. Charlie signed and started to get up and leave.

"Hold on a second, Dad. You've got to sign your own card," Mikey said.

"I just signed," said Charlie.

"You signed Dan's card."

"Who's Dan?" asked Charlie.

"That's Dan Morres, Dad," Mikey said, motioning toward Dan.

Dan Morres really shot himself out of the tournament in the first round and wasn't likely to make the cut, walked up to Charlie and stuck out his hand for a hand shake. "Charlie, I'm Dan Morres and I want to tell you that it was really a pleasure playing golf with you yesterday and today. The putt you made today on eleven was the very best putt I've ever witnessed. You are my favorite to win this tournament. Play well," he said as he turned his card in and walked out of the tent.

Mikey got Charlie's score card from Bob Gilder and reviewed the hole by hole scores. It was correct so he handed it to Charlie and said, "Here's your card, Dad. Sign it and we'll turn it in."

"Okay," replied Charlie as he took the card, signed it in the correct spot and handed it to the official in the tent.

They soon had everything done in the scoring tent and were ready to head to the locker room to change Charlie's shoes. As they walked out of the tent, they encountered a sea of reporters, each trying to get the one interview from Charlie, the golfer with Alzheimer's.

CBS crews were televising the tournament during the weekend. They also provided the most money to the USGA so they now had priority for interviews, even if it was a day before they officially began covering the tournament. The interview was with Brent Musberger and it was his task was to get an interview with Charlie Caldwell. "Charlie," Brent called out. "Can we have a few words with you?" he asked.

"Okay," replied Charlie.

Brent led Charlie toward a special area that had been roped off for CBS's use only and using the back drop of the beautiful club house. Brent began the interview by making sure Charlie was comfortable before they began filming.

Before the questions began, Mikey tried to intervene so he could help his father answer difficult questions. Before he could get by his father's side, Brent said, "Mikey, let's try the interview with just Charlie."

"Dad will not be able to answer many of your questions, Mister Musberger," replied Mikey. "We've tried this before and it just doesn't work well."

"Mikey, stay close and if we need you, you'll be called to come forward. I've completed interviews like this before and think I can make everyone happy."

Mikey was forced to stay on the sidelines of the interview, and he simply said "Okay."

Brent got the cue from the camera man and began the interview with a basic introduction. "Charlie Caldwell just finished the second round and ended up with a two over par seventy-three. And folks, that is despite beginning the round with a disastrous eight on the first hole. His total for the two days is two-under par. Many of you may have heard Charlie's name before as he almost won the 1978 US Open. He took an amazing twelve strokes on the last hole of that tournament to move from a tie for first to finishing in a dismal tie for fourteenth."

"Charlie, does your start in this year's Senior Open remind you of your performance in the 1978 Open?" asked Brent.

Charlie looked at Brent and then the camera for a few seconds. He looked back at Brent again and responded, "I don't know."

Brent knew at this point the interview would be a bit more difficult than he thought. He decided to keep the questions simple. "Charlie, you were leading the tournament yesterday with an outstanding sixty-seven. You had a couple of great holes out there yesterday and Bob Gilder was one of your playing partners for the first two rounds. Bob described your shot on eleven yesterday as being one of the very best he's ever seen. What club did you use yesterday?" Brent asked.

"I can't remember," replied Charlie quickly.

"Okay, you can't remember. We looked at the film and it looks like you used an older fairway wood. We're going to ask your caddie to bring that club in so the folks at home can see this club. As he gets the club, let's go over your shot on that hole today."

Mikey hurried off to get the celebrated five-wood and really felt he should not have left Charlie alone with the CBS crew. He made it very quick.

Charlie watched Mikey leave the area and turned back toward Brent. "Okay," replied Charlie.

"We're you trying to make birdie on eleven, or were you just trying to two-putt for a par?" Brent asked.

"I'm sorry, I can't remember. Did I make par?" Charlie asked.

"No, you made birdie today and that gives you two straight on this difficult par-three. Many of the golfers have described it as the toughest par-three on the tour," replied Brent. "Are you serious, Charlie? You cannot remember what you hit on that hole?"

"My memory is not very good anymore. The doctor's think that I have some disease. I forget the name, but I don't believe them. I just have a hard time remembering things," replied Charlie.

Mikey came back with the five-wood and it was handed to Brent.

"We have the five-wood that Charlie Caldwell used to make birdie on the eleventh hole yesterday and again today. It is an older wooden club and I believe it's the only wooden five-wood used by any professional golfer playing on the tour this year." Holding the club up so viewers could see Charlie and club at the same time, he added a question, "Charlie, what is special about this club?"

"I don't know," replied Charlie. "It looks just like one of the golf clubs that Diane bought for me."

"Diane? Is Diane your wife, Charlie?"

Charlie looked puzzled and replied very quietly, "Yes, I think so. Mikey is my caddie and he knows for sure. Ask Mikey," he added.

Brent finally had enough of Charlie's lack of ability to answer questions and called for Mikey to join. "Mikey, your father is not able to answer a lot of questions. Can you help us understand what's going through his mind?"

"I'll be glad to try and help," replied Mikey.

"Does your father know that he has Alzheimer's?" asked Brent.

Charlie heard the word and suddenly replied quite loudly, "That's the name of the thing they say I have."

Mikey intervened with Charlie. "Yes, Dad. That is what they say you have, but they don't know for sure, huh?"

"No, they are stupid," said Charlie in a much softer tone this time.

Charlie looked at Brent and softly said, "Mister Musburger, my father does not like to hear people say he has Alzheimer's. As you can see, he can get pretty vocal about it too. We have found that he doesn't get nearly as upset if you just refer to him having memory problems."

Brent nodded approval to Mikey. "We will not use that term again," he said. "Your father knows that he has a memory problem but he does not think the problem is from a disease. He just thinks he has a memory problem, just like most people have in their later years. The doctors have also not been able to positively say he has the disease either."

"How does he cope with memory problems on the course? Can he remember his score after playing a hole?" Brent asked.

"Sometimes he can, but quite often he can't even remember his last shot."

"That seems like it would be very difficult for you as a son, let alone for you as a caddie. How do you cope with your father's disease or memory problem?"

145

"That's really simple. I let him be a golfer hitting one shot at a time. I figure out the distance and based upon that, I give my father a particular golf club and tell him where to hit it," replied Mikey. "He may not know what he did on the last shot and usually has problems remembering how far he can hit certain clubs. However, if you give him the right club and tell him where he should hit the golf ball, he'll amaze you time after time. At least, it certainly amazes me."

"You gave your father the five-wood to hit on ten and eleven yesterday. He also birdied the par three on both days. Did he surprise you with those shots?"

"Actually, I wanted him to hit an iron short of the green on ten yesterday, but he wanted to go for it. You do not want to be long on that hole, because if goes down over the green and down the hill, you almost guaranteed to be in the hazard. He seemed to be pretty confident yesterday so I let him go for it with the five-wood. You saw the result. He hit a great shot that ended up on the green from an almost impossible location. His five-wood almost went in on the par three eleventh," Mikey said.

"Yes, it was a super shot. Let's talk about Charlie's play on that hole today," Brent added. "Charlie hit the same five-wood today but he was considerably short."

"Actually, it was almost the same distance and the flight of the ball was similar too. The only difference was that the greens were a bit softer today. Yesterday's shot hit and ran forward and today's stopped within inches of the ball mark. But what about his putt today?" Mikey added. "I estimated the double break on his putt on eleven and pointed to the line I wanted him to hit. Dad's putt actually stopped before something caused it to wobble and it turned toward the hole. We were lucky it hit the hole too. If it wouldn't have hit the hole, he would have had ten to fifteen feet coming back."

"Yeah, we were all watching it. I have witnessed thousands of putts in my years of covering golf and I must say, that was the highlight of all of them," Brent said. "Okay, Mikey, let's talk about the start today. Charlie made an eight on the hole. Was he nervous following his great round from yesterday?"

"Dad was a bit nervous on the first tee for sure. It wasn't about being in the Senior Open though. He really doesn't understand that he is playing in a major tournament and that's not what affected him today. I saw a hesitation in his set up and stepped in. He stopped his swing and told me that he was afraid of missing his shot and hitting one of the spectators with the golf ball. I tried to reassure him but it was still in his mind when he finally hit the ball. Normally he has a very slow and methodical swing but this morning it was not smooth. He failed to finish the swing and you saw the result. It was a low ball that barely cleared the fans on the right side of the tee box. That was the reason for him being a bit nervous on the first tee. It wasn't because this was the US Senior Open."

"This is the biggest senior event in golf. How does he not know that he's actually playing in the tournament?" asked Brent.

"I have no idea," replied Mikey. "But he doesn't."

"It looks like you're going to be a couple of shots out of the lead when it comes to Saturday's round. Is there anything you plan to do to help your dad prepare?" asked Brent.

"I'd love to let him sleep in but he's usually asleep by nine and almost always up before six," replied Mikey. "Of course, if he's awake, I have to be awake to watch him. If I turn my head for one minute, he could be gone on his next adventure. Getting back to your question of what we're doing to prepare for tomorrow's round. We really won't do anything out of the ordinary. As far as my dad knows, he will be playing golf with another golfer."

Brent looked like he was intently following Mikey's conversation and smiled softly as Mikey finished. "Thank you, Mikey," he said. Turning toward Charlie, Brent concluded the interview with, "Charlie Caldwell, best of luck tomorrow and thanks for the opportunity to let everyone know a little bit about you."

As if on cue, Charlie looked at the camera and just smiled softly and said, "Okay."

The director in the control booth watched this and realized it would be one of the most noteworthy finishes ever for a golf interview. "Wow!" he said out loud. "That was precious!"

The camera light went off and a technician removed the pinned-on lapel microphone from Charlie's shirt.

Mikey put Charlie's club back in the bag and the two again headed for the club house. There was a continual flood of people asking Charlie to sign anything and everything. Charlie was getting to be pretty good at signing his signature but did not have the slightest idea why people were asking for it.

Finally, they made it through the clubhouse and quickly got in the car that had been pulled up for a quick getaway. They headed directly for the hotel. As they pulled into the parking area, several reporters from other news sources and papers ran up trying to get their own interview. Mikey declined them all and did not answer any of their questions. Soon, the two were in the seclusion of their own room in the DoubleTree.

Chapter Eleven

Saturday was like the other days they spent in Rochester. They were up early and Charlie had his usual pancakes and also added a waffle today. After breakfast, they went back to the room for a while before heading to the golf course to get ready to play a round of golf.

They were in the room when Diane called. Friday's round was televised, but was on a cable channel that she didn't have so she didn't any idea how well Charlie was playing until she called some friends.

The call came as a pleasant surprise for Charlie and when Mikey said, "Dad, Mom's on the phone and she wants to talk to you," When Charlie realized it was Diane on the phone, he giggled like a child getting ready to open gifts at Christmas.

"Yes, yes... Hello Diane. Are you here now?" he asked.

"No, Charlie, I'm still in San Antonio but I wish I would have flown to Rochester with you and Mikey now. I read the newspaper this morning and they said that you started off kind of shaky yesterday but really pulled it together later on. I'm so proud of you, Charlie."

"Yeah," said Charlie. "We played golf yesterday and I think we will be playing golf today."

He paused for a second or two and added, "Diane, people really like to watch golf up here. There are lots of people that watch us play golf. I don't know why they don't play too but I guess they just like to watch people play golf."

"They are watching you play golf, Charlie," said Diane. "You're one of the best golfers in the world and people really like to watch you play."

"Nah, they're not just watching me. They watch everybody else, too. But, you know what?" he added.

"No, what?" she asked.

"They call out my name all the time. They say, Charlie… Charlie. I don't know why they are always calling out my name, but Mikey tells me to smile and wave at the people."

"Yes, I saw that on television today. ESPN had a report on you and they said that almost all of the people were shouting out 'Charlie… Charlie.' They showed a clip of you making a birdie on number eleven and when the putt went in, everyone seemed to be yelling your name. They also said that it could be heard all over the golf course, too. That must have been exciting, huh?" she asked.

"Yeah, it was cool," replied Charlie.

They talked for a few more minutes and Diane had to break the conversation as Charlie would have talked to her all day long.

Charlie was in the third from the final group and was scheduled to tee off at two-forty in the afternoon so they had some time to kill. Mikey looked at the clock on the night stand and realized they had almost six hours before it was time to head to the course. He knew keeping Charlie's mind occupied for several hours in a hotel room would be impossible.

It was just after nine in the morning and Mikey realized that the mall would probably be open. "Hey Dad, let's go to the mall and buy something for Mom."

"Okay," replied Charlie.

Mikey checked with the concierge at the hotel and was directed to a mall that was on the way to the country club. He thought that would be a good place for the two of them to kill a couple of hours.

Soon, they were in the car and making the short drive from the DoubleTree. As they were pulling into the mall, Charlie noticed that there was a golf store too. "Mikey," he said. "There's a golf store here. Let's go."

"Okay, we'll make sure we go by the golf store. Are you looking for something special?"

"No, I just like looking at all the new stuff."

They stopped by several stores looking for something for Diane but didn't really find anything special. Charlie wanted to buy everything he saw for Diane, but everything he suggested was something he liked but wouldn't necessarily be what Diane wanted.

They were going through a Sharper Image and both agreed that Diane would like an electronic picture frame. Charlie really liked it but Mikey realized that he actually liked almost everything he saw. Taking his dad shopping was much like taking a five year old shopping. They want to buy everything and have little or no concern why they want something or how much it costs.

Mikey took the electronic picture frame from Charlie and said, "Mom will really like this, Dad. You made a great choice."

"Okay," replied Charlie.

As they left the Sharper Image store, they turned right and there was the golf store that Charlie saw while in the car. "Hey Mikey, there's the golf store. Let's go look and see what they have."

"Okay, let's do that," replied Mikey.

They walked into the store and down the aisles of clubs, shoes, bags and other apparel. They were at the back of the store when Charlie noticed the indoor driving range where customers could test clubs before they made their purchase. Charlie selected a driver from the selection and walked into the driving cage. This cage was fully automated with the latest technology.

Charlie took the driver and looked down at the ball that was resting on the rubber tee. He took a slow practice swing and then moved up to address. Charlie repeated the same swing and sent the ball travelling on the perfect trajectory. As soon as he hit the ball, the rubber tee dropped down and then appeared with a new ball.

Charlie was flabbergasted. "Mikey," he yelled. "You gotta see this. I hit the ball and this thing puts another ball on the tee. We got to get one of these things."

Mikey had not seen anything like this either. "This is really cool, Dad. We should get one of these so you can practice more, huh?"

"Okay," replied Charlie as he continued to hit the driver into the net.

The two didn't notice but someone apparently recognized Charlie from the tournament and soon there were dozens of people standing behind the practice area watching Charlie hit the driver.

After hitting one of the shots, Charlie turned and saw all the people. Like he was taught by Mikey, he made a soft wave of the hand. He then turned back and watched the rubber tee move down and retrieve another ball.

Mikey noticed the other people now and was a bit nervous. He assumed they may be waiting to try their clubs on the practice area. "Oh, we're sorry. Are you waiting to use the range?" he asked.

"No, we're just watching Mister Caldwell hit the driver," one of the people said. "He has a real good swing."

"Well, we're just killing some time before our tee time this afternoon. Dad was intrigued with how the balls keep popping up on the rubber things. We're about through here though. We'll kill another hour or so, have lunch then head out to Oak Hill," said Mikey. "Are you guys going to watch the tournament today?"

One of the group answered first, "Tickets for the weekend are pretty hard to get. I had tickets for Thursday and Friday but wasn't able to get tickets for the weekend."

Mikey realized that each golfer in the tournament had a series of tickets that were reserved for the golfer's friends or family. "Guys, I think we have access to ten free passes and we have only used one so far. If you give me a list of names, I'll drop the list off at the call window and you can watch the tournament today and tomorrow."

"That will be great," one said as he looked around to the other people standing in the group.

Mikey got the names of everyone as Charlie kept hitting drivers into the net. Soon, he had all the information he needed and looked at Charlie. "Dad, let's grab some lunch and then head to the course. I don't want to see you tire yourself out too quick."

"Okay," replied Charlie as he set the club down.

The two had lunch in the mall and then headed to the course. Mikey dropped the list of names off at the USGA tournament office and they assured him that tickets would be available for those people.

With that issue resolved, the two worked their way through the crowd of fans with Charlie again signing hundreds of autographs. With the help of the security team that finally showed up, they found themselves on the protected ground of the club house.

As they were making their way to the practice area, Abe caught up with them. Charlie saw Abe as he was walking up to them and said, "Abe, are you going to caddie for me today?"

"No, Charlie. You have your son, Mikey on the bag today. He's doing a great job too," replied Abe.

"But Abe, you have been my caddie for a long time. Why aren't you going to caddie for me today?"

Abe looked at Charlie and then Mikey. "Charlie," he said, "Mikey is the best caddie in the world and you need him on the bag."

Mikey intervened and added, "Dad, Abe was going to caddie but his back is giving him problems. Let me carry your bag, Okay?"

"Well, I guess," replied Charlie.

Charlie was suddenly caught up with signing autographs again and Abe took the time to speak with Mikey. "Mikey, I seem to be causing your father some problems today. I don't want to do anything that breaks his concentration on what you're telling him to do."

Mikey looked at Abe and said, "That's not true Abe. You are one of dad's best friends and he needs you to be by his side."

"No, Mikey, he does not need me. He has his son by his side and that is the perfect combination. I'll still be there but will be on the sidelines. If you listen close, you will hear me yell too."

Mikey started to respond but Abe raised his hand. "Mikey, that is the way it is. You stay by Charlie's side and remember, I'll be there cheering you on."

"Okay," responded Mikey as he watched Abe leave and make his way back to the course.

Mikey rescued his father from all the autograph seekers and they finally made it to the protection of the driving range. Like each of the previous days on the driving range, Charlie was again amazed that they had new Titleist range balls to hit. "Mikey, these are all new balls," he said with the same excitement in his voice.

Mikey looked at his father and repeated his response from the previous days. "Dad, these are brand new balls! They have brand new balls on the driving range. This is a high-class place, huh?"

"Yeah, it is a nice driving range for sure," replied Charlie.

There were a couple of thousand fans maneuvering for the best view on the driving range and Mikey looked back to see that most were trying to get the perfect angle to watch Charlie in his warm-up routine.

Charlie hit the one hundred yard sign on his third wedge, which brought on some loud clapping from the fans that were watching from the gallery. He again hit the sign a few shots later and the clapping was louder this time.

Mikey realized that the clapping could be disturbing to the other golfers so he took the wedge and handed Charlie the nine-iron. He knew that this club would go past the sign and therefore wouldn't create any disturbance with the other golfers.

After hitting balls, the two were escorted by security teams to the practice putting green where Charlie showed that he was still in fine form with the flat stick. He made all of the three-footers and all but one of the putts from five feet.

Mikey liked what he saw in his father today. He was very relaxed but enjoying the crowds. Hopefully, they would get off the first tee with a good shot and continue solid play throughout the round.

Eventually, they were called to the tee where their playing partner, Jay Hass, was already there talking with the starter.

Mikey set the bag down and walked with Charlie to the starter where he introduced his father to Jay Hass. "Mister Hass, this is my father, Charlie Caldwell."

Jay shook Charlie's hand and said, "Hello Charlie. I've been following your play this week and it's outstanding. Let's have an enjoyable round."

Charlie shook Jay's hand and replied, "Okay."

Charlie looked at Mikey and asked, "Where's the guy that we played with before?"

"We played with Bob Gilder before but he's already gone off. We're playing with someone new today. His name is Jay Hass."

"Okay," replied Charlie.

Jay was the first to go off and the starter called him to the box. "Ladies and Gentlemen, playing from St. Louis, Missouri, PGA Professional Jay Hass."

Jay walked to the tee, placed a ball on the tee and drove it long and straight down the middle.

The crowd clapped loudly and Jay acknowledge with a wave.

Charlie watched Jay's ball and remarked to Mikey, "That was a real long shot. Did you see how far that fella hit the ball?"

"Yes, I did. He is one of the longest hitters for sure. He may be longer than you but you're much more accurate. Let's just hit our regular shot down the middle. Aim for the center of the fairway," Mikey said.

"Okay," replied Charlie.

The starter called Charlie to the tee. "Ladies and Gentlemen, playing out of San Antonio, Texas, please welcome PGA Professional Charlie Caldwell."

The crowd clapped loudly and Charlie acknowledged with a small wave.

He placed a ball on the tee, took the one practice swing and drove the ball down the middle and at least fifty yards short of Jay Hass' ball.

157

The tees were further back today and Charlie's drive left him about one hundred and seventy yards from the flag. Mikey measured the distance and looked where the pin placement sheet had placed the flag. It was exactly one hundred and seventy-six yards to the hole.

Mikey knew that his dad hit the six-iron one hundred and seventy yards and hit the five-iron one hundred and eighty-two yards on the fly. Rather than having his father try to shorten the distance of the five-iron, Mikey elected to have him hit the solid six-iron to the center of the green. He handed his father the six-iron.

"Dad, aim at the center of the green," he said.

Charlie took the six-iron and took the one practice swing before hitting a solid shot that flew exactly one hundred and seventy-four yards. The ball took one bounce and stopped two feet from the hole.

"Nice shot, Charlie," said Jay Hass. "That's the way to start the round."

"Okay," replied Charlie.

Jay's ball was almost as good a shot but the wedge put a lot of spin on the ball, causing it to back up some fifteen feet from the hole.

Jay two-putted for his par and Charlie easily made his putt for birdie.

After he tapped the ball in, the crowd began the chant "Charlie… Charlie…." To which, Charlie simply waved his hand.

Both golfers made par on the second and third holes. Charlie was still up first when they came to the reachable par-five, on the front side. Charlie's ball was down the middle but he was still over three hundred yards away from the green. However, Jay's tee shot was extra-long and he only had about two hundred and forty yards to the pin.

Mikey handed his father the five-wood and gave directions to go down the middle, which he did perfectly. It left him with an easy wedge to the flag.

Jay used a hybrid and reached the right-side of the green, leaving him with a fairly lengthy eagle putt.

As they walked to Charlie's ball, Mikey measured the exact distance. It was almost exactly one hundred yards to the flag. He handed the wedge to his father and gave instructions to aim directly at the flag. Charlie took the one practice swing and then hit a perfectly timed shot. It hit a yard short of the flag, took one bounce and disappeared. Mikey thought at first that it went over the green but Charlie knew it was in the hole. "That went in, Mikey," he said.

It was confirmed when Mikey saw the acknowledgement from Jay Hass and then from the crowd. It got louder and louder as the two walked up to the green and Charlie walked to the flag and retrieved the ball.

The chant now seemed like it was coming from all over. Even fans on other holes seemed to be shouting the chant. As soon as the three was recorded on the scoreboard near the clubhouse, those fans joined in to the chant.

As Charlie and Mikey walked up to the green, they noticed that even Jay Hass was clapping and shouting, "Charlie... Charlie."

Jay held out his fist as Charlie walked by and was presented with a fist bump from the eagle maker.

It was now time for Jay to putt and Mikey raised his arms to quiet the crowd and the loud roar suddenly quieted. The silence was noticeable as Jay studied the putt from all angles. Soon, he had the line and made what he called his best putt of the tournament. The twenty-footer was in all the way and when it also found the bottom of the hole, the quiet again erupted in a deafening uproar.

Charlie now held out his fist to Jay who promptly returned the fist bump.

Charlie was three under for the round going into the long par three eleventh and Jay had dropped one shot to be one under.

Mikey studied the pin sheet and determined the exact yardage to the pin was just over two hundred yards. He handed Charlie the same five-wood that he used to make birdie on Thursday and Friday. Charlie used the five-wood and repeated the same swing that was successful days before. The ball landed about ten feet from the pin, leaving Charlie an uphill and fairly straight putt.

Jay hit his shot and was pin-high just left of the green. His chip was within inches and he tapped in for his par.

Mikey looked at the putt and determined that there was not enough break to aim outside of the hole. He looked at his father and noticed that Charlie had a very nervous look on his face. Charlie was also grimacing like something was causing him pain. Mikey knew something was wrong, real wrong.

Momentarily forgetting about the putt, Mikey quickly made his way to Charlie's side. "What's the matter, Dad?" he asked.

"Mikey, I think I made a mess," he said almost crying. "I really made a mess, Mikey."

"How did you make a mess?" Mikey asked before immediately recognizing from the odor what the mess was.

"Dad, did you make a mess in your pants?" he asked.

"Yes, I pooped my pants," he answered very quietly. "I tried to hold it but I couldn't."

"Dad, wait right here. I'm going to get your rain pants and then get you cleaned up."

"Okay," said Charlie.

Mikey ran over to Jay Haas and said, "Jay, my father just had an accident and crapped in his pants. I have got to take him to one of the bathroom facilities on the course."

Jay Haas rolled his eyes and said, "This is unbelievable."

Mikey didn't hear Jay's comment and quickly went over to the USGA official that was following the group. "Sir, my father has just had an accident and crapped in his pants. We need to get him to a bathroom so he can get cleaned up."

"What are you going to do? We don't have enough time to go back to the clubhouse. You will have to use one of the bathrooms near the green on number eight," he said quickly. "You can use a golf cart for this so I'll have one sent out."

"Okay, I'll get dad's rain pants and we should be back on the course in a few minutes," Mikey said as he went to get his father and some rain pants out of the bag.

"Dad, let's go," Mikey said as he grabbed the rain pants out of the bag. He had them and they quickly walked to where the USGA official was standing, still on the radio.

He finished his conversation on the radio and said to Mikey, "They are ruling this as a medical emergency and you have ten minutes to either fix the issue or you will be disqualified."

"Okay, I think we can make it," Mikey said as the golf cart quickly arrived.

Mikey and Charlie got on and they were quickly taken to the rest room facility near the green on number eight. Luckily, a local marshal cleared the restroom so Mikey and Charlie had it all to themselves.

"Hurry, Dad. Take off your shoes and take down your pants," Mikey said.

Charlie used his feet to take off his shoes and then dropped his trousers.

"Mikey saw the mess and said, "Oh, my God. This is not going to be fun. Dad, why didn't you say you had to go to the bathroom?"

"I didn't think about it until I couldn't wait. I'm sorry, Mikey," he added. "I tried to hold it."

Mikey took his father's underwear off and grabbed some paper towels. He wiped off shit from Charlie's butt and legs, while wincing from the odor.

Within a few minutes, he had his father respectably cleaned up. Luckily, he had the rain pants as the regular trousers were beyond cleaning. Mikey, rolled the messy trousers and underwear and put them into the trash can.

162

"Here, Dad. Put on these rain pants," he said. "We need to be quick as we're running out of time."

Charlie had a look of fear on his face. "Mikey, I don't want to go back out there. This is embarrassing and everyone will know I just shit in my pants. Let's stay here until it's dark, then go home."

"Dad, the people don't know that you had an accident. They just think that you had to go to the bathroom. Don't worry about it," Mikey added, trying to reassure his father.

Charlie had the rain pants on and quickly slipped into his golf shoes.

They both used toilet paper to clean their hands and then ran out where the marshal was holding back a large crowd.

"What happened?" some of the fans asked.

Mikey looked at one of the fans and simply said, "Medical emergency."

Within eight minutes, they were back by the eleventh green. Jay Haas was still standing near the area where golfers would be walking to the next tee.

"Is everything Okay?" he asked.

"Yeah, it's fine now," replied Mikey.

The official was just getting off the radio informing the groups behind that everything was corrected in time and they would be finishing the hole in a moment.

Mikey handed the putter to his father and reviewed the situation. He looked at the green and determined the slope. His instruction to Charlie was to aim at the center and hit it firm. Charlie followed the instructions perfectly and knocked the putt firmly in the hole for the third consecutive birdie on this difficult par-three.

As soon as the putt fell in to the hole, Charlie smiled. He didn't wave to the crowd as he may have still been embarrassed by what just happened. Jay looked at Charlie and said, "Nice birdie."

Charlie didn't even acknowledge Jay's comment.

Mikey looked at his dad and realized that his dad recovered from a situation that would have destroyed most people. "How embarrassing it would be to crap your pants in front of thousands of people standing around you and millions watching on the television," Mikey thought to himself.

However, Mikey thought that having Alzheimer's could be a blessing to someone who forgot that it was only a few minutes earlier when he shit his pants in front of the world. Those moments were now buried forever and Charlie was back having the time of his life. It made Mikey feel very good inside.

Charlie had one additional birdie on the back nine and carded a five under par round for the day and that left him at seven under par for the entire tournament. Mikey looked at the scoreboard and saw that his dad was now leading the tournament with a two shot lead over Tom Watson and Bernard Langer.

Mikey escorted Charlie into the scorer's tent and exchanged cards with Jay. Together they went over each golfer's score hole by hole. Mikey checked every hole twice and totaled the round before handing it to his father to sign. Charlie signed the card with a simple "Charlie" and handed it to the official scorer.

Jay verified his card and also handed it to the score after signing. Jay turned to Charlie and shook his hand once again. "Charlie, it was my distinct pleasure playing golf with you today. You are a very special person and it was spectacular watching you hit some of the shots you pulled off today. As far as I'm concerned, this round playing with you was the highlight for me during the tournament. Thank you for allowing me to be part of this day, this very special day."

Jay started to walk outside and again turned back to Charlie and Mikey. "By the way, you guys handled the situation on eleven perfectly. I would still be in the bathroom hiding."

Charlie looked at Mikey and asked, "What happened on eleven?"

"Nothing happened on eleven, Dad. You just made another birdie," Mikey said.

"Oh, Okay," Charlie replied.

Mikey escorted Charlie out of the scorer's tent and into the throng of people that were all waiting for Charlie. They all were still chanting, "Charlie... Charlie." The security people realized that their services were required and forcibly maneuvered their way to Charlie and Mikey to form a walkway from the scorer's tent to the clubhouse. Charlie was all smiles as he made the walk and was fist pumping everyone who stuck out their hand.

Brent Musburger was there and again wanted to interview Charlie. This time Mikey was with Charlie and answered most of the questions. Mikey also told them that he was not going to answer any questions concerning the incident that took place on eleven today.

"Charlie Caldwell had another fantastic round today and is here with us. Today was an excellent display of golf, Charlie. You seem to be in control the entire day and really you were never in trouble. Did you do anything different this morning or last night to help you with your golf game?" asked Musburger.

"Today was fun," replied Charlie. "People were shouting my name all the time and sometimes it was so loud it hurt my ears. Did you hear the people shouting, 'Charlie... Charlie'?" He asked.

"Yes, we heard that all day and it was not just around the hole that you are playing, but it seemed to come from everywhere on the golf course," replied Musburger. "But let's get back to the question I asked earlier. Did you do anything special this morning to prepare you for shooting such a great score today?"

Mikey stepped in as he realized his father would not be able to answer this question. "Dad did not do anything special this morning. We were both out of bed around 6:30am and had a leisurely breakfast. Dad had his favorite breakfast, which is a pancake with maple syrup. After breakfast we walked around the mall for a while and stopped in a local golf store where he hit a few drives with different clubs. After that, we came straight to the golf course and went through our regular routine for warming up. He putted for a few minutes before starting around with Jay Haas. And I must say that dad really enjoyed playing with Jay today. Jay had two spectacular shots to get on the green and had a great putt for an eagle. Dad does not have the length to have reached the green in two so I had him lay-up. He had a 100 yard shot to the pin. He pulled off the perfect shot and the ball landed short of the pin, took two hops and then disappeared into the hole. With Jay also scoring and eagle three everyone was having a great time."

"Well Charlie, it looks like it will be you and Tom Watson playing together tomorrow. The last group is still on the course, but it does look like you and Watson will be in the final group. From what we understand you have never had the opportunity to play up with Tom Watson. Are you nervous going into the last round playing with someone who has won this tournament three times before?" asked Musburger.

"No," replied Charlie.

Mikey realized that the answer would not be enough to satisfy Musburger so he again stepped in. "Dad doesn't really get nervous anymore," replied Mikey. "He is simply playing golf without realizing who he is playing with or which tournament it is. To him it's just like he's going out and playing a Sunday round."

Musburger appeared to be a little irritated and cut Mikey off. "Before we get back to the tournament, Charlie, I want to tell you that we have received thousands of e-mails about your performance so far this week. Everyone wishes you the best of luck in tomorrow's final round. Good luck and like everybody else around Oak Hill country club, most of the country will be shouting 'Charlie... Charlie,' with the rest of the crowd, tomorrow."

Brent Musburger turned back toward the camera and said, "Let's get back to the 18th where Greg Norman is finishing."

That concluded the interview so Charlie and Mikey left and walked through the crowd to the clubhouse. Charlie changed shoes and the two walked to the car that one of the attendants delivered. They were soon off the grounds of the country club and headed back to the hotel.

As they drive up to the DoubleTree, Mikey noticed all of the news trucks and reporters waiting in the parking lot. "Holy cow, there are hundreds of reporters waiting for us," Mikey said quietly. "Dad, getting through that crowd of reporters will be impossible. Let's find a new place to stay tonight?" Mikey asked without expecting a reply.

Charlie didn't reply as usual. He simply grunted, "ughh."

Mikey was not sure where he was going he just continued to drive away from the DoubleTree. After driving several miles he sees a sign for Best Western Motel and pulls into the parking lot. He and Charlie go to the front desk and book a room for the evening.

Fortunately the room was on the ground floor and they were able to park right in front of the door. Mikey and Charlie got out of the car and quickly went into the room. Mikey locked the door and Charlie went straight for the television, which he turned on.

Mikey grabbed the remote and turned the television off. "Dad, you have got to take a shower. You had an accident on the golf course today and need to get cleaned up. Let's get the shower set up for you so you can get cleaned up."

Charlie realized that he did smell and agreed to take a shower without arguing. He quickly took off his clothes and got into the shower that Mikey had set up. Mikey stood outside the shower to make sure he cleaned himself.

Since Charlie didn't have anything else to wear, Mikey turned the rain pants inside-out and helped his father get in them.

Mikey turned the television back on and tossed the remote to Charlie.

Charlie lied back on the bed and began flipping the channels. Charlie finally stopped flipping when he came upon a National Geographic or Animal Planet show that had lions or crocodiles killing wildebeests. These were Charlie's favorite shows to watch and they can occupy him for hours on end.

Charlie had himself propped up on the bed while Mikey took the other one. Soon Charlie said started bobbing up and down and he began to snore softly.

Mikey looked at his dad and thought about waking him up so they could go get something to eat and buy him some fresh clothes to wear for tomorrow's final round. After watching his dad sleep for a minute or so, Mikey thought he could get away and only be gone for a few minutes at the most. His dad would never know that he was gone. Something told him that this was not the right move, but he preferred not to wake him. Mikey quietly got off the bed and left the room without waking Charlie.

He started the car and drove out the parking lot and down the road toward the Wal-Mart that was in the next block. His plan was to buy the clothes that Charlie would need tomorrow, a razor, two toothbrushes and some toothpaste before stopping by McDonald's on the way back.

Chapter Twelve

Mikey arrived back at the motel room and immediately knew something was wrong as the door to the room was open. He hadn't been gone for more than thirty to forty minutes. If Charlie left the room, he couldn't have gone far, Mikey thought. Mikey checked the bathroom, pulled back the shower curtain and still no Charlie. Mikey quickly walked out of the room leaving the door open just in case Charlie returned. He walked to the office of the motel and asked if anyone had seen in elderly man walking by. Of course, the answer was no.

Mikey ran out to the road and quickly looked to the right and to the left. Again, he did not see Charlie.

He ran back to the office and used the office phone to call Nine-One-One. "Nine-One-One, what is your emergency please?" asked the operator.

"Yes, this is Michael Caldwell, and I would like to report a missing person," replied Mikey.

"All right Sir, we will get on the case right away but first I need to get some additional information," said the operator. "What is your name again?"

"Michael Caldwell," replied Mikey.

"What is your location and what is your phone number just in case we get cut off?" She asked.

"I am calling on the Best Western motel and we're located on South Clover Street., just south of Rochester. I don't know the phone number but I can get it from the office if you need it."

"If we get cut off, I can get the phone number fairly easy. Okay, what is the name of the missing person?"

"The missing person is my father and his name is Charlie Caldwell. He is 56 years old and is suffering from Alzheimer's. We need to find him quickly, as he is playing in the US Senior golf tournament open tomorrow," replied Mikey.

"All right Sir, how long has Charlie been missing?"

"He's been missing for about an hour now."

"One hour. We do not usually begin a missing person's investigation until the person has been missing for 24 hours, Sir."

"But ma'am, you don't understand. My father, Charlie Caldwell, has early stages of Alzheimer's and has no idea where he is at, or how to get back to the motel. We have to find him quickly so he can make his tee time tomorrow afternoon," replied Mikey as he began to get a little agitated with the operator.

"Sir, if I understand this right, you want us to try and find your father so he can make a tee time tomorrow. Is that correct?" She asked.

"Yes ma'am. That is what I'm asking."

"That does not meet our requirements for beginning a missing person's investigation, Sir. Your father is probably somewhere around the motel and will probably return on his own. However, if he doesn't turn by tomorrow afternoon, call us back and we will begin the investigation at that time."

"Ma'am, I cannot wait until tomorrow to find him. May I speak to your supervisor?" Mikey asked.

"Yes, Sir, please hold the line and I will get Sergeant Washington on the phone."

Mikey had to wait a few minutes but eventually Sergeant Washington came on the phone. "Good evening, this is Sergeant Washington of the Rochester Police Department. I understand your father has been missing for about an hour and you want to initiate a missing persons report. Is that correct Sir?"

"Yes sir. That is exactly what I want. Sergeant Washington, do you play golf or have you been following the US Senior open golf tournament going on in Rochester this week?" Mikey asked.

"No sir, I am not into golf but I am aware of the golf tournament going on this week. We have several patrolmen on security detail at the country club. As a matter of fact, one of them is on duty with me at the moment."

"Sir, ask that patrolman if he's heard of Charlie Caldwell."

"Okay Sir just a moment," replied Sergeant Washington.

Mikey could hear the Sergeant ask the patrolman if he heard of his father. "Hey Barry, have you heard of Charlie Caldwell?"

Mikey could not hear the response from the patrolman but Barry soon came on the line. "Sir, are you saying that the missing person is the same Charlie Caldwell that's playing in the Open?"

"Yes Sir that is exactly what I'm saying. My name is Michael Caldwell and I am his son as well as his caddie. As you probably have heard, he has second stage Alzheimer's. He somehow got away from me at the hotel and he probably has

172

no idea of where he's at. He could be anywhere within this area. We need to find him as soon as possible," replied Mikey.

"Okay sir, I'll make sure that we get the case opened up immediately. I see on the report that you're staying at the Best Western motel on Clover Street. We will have somebody there within 15 minutes. What was your father wearing when you last saw him?" asked the patrolman.

"He was wearing the same thing that he wore in the tournament today. He had on golfing rain pants and a light blue golf shirt. He had a pullover but that is in the room now, so all he has on is the rain pants and a light blue shirt."

"Okay, where was Charlie at when you last saw him?"

"Charlie was lying on the bed in the room," replied Mikey.

"Michael, why didn't you stay at the DoubleTree with most of the other golfers?" asked Officer Johnson.

"We were staying there but when we left the country club this afternoon to drive back to the DoubleTree, I saw all the press vehicles at our motel. The media coverage on my father causes too much stress on him so I drove on and decided to find another place to stay for the night. That is how we ended up at the Best Western. We got in the room around 7:30pm, and dad lay down on the bed. He was exhausted and he fell asleep within minutes. I knew that I had to run to the store to get him some clothes to wear tomorrow and to get some other stuff for us for the evening. I thought about waking him up but knew that I was only going to be gone for a few minutes since Wal-Mart is right down the road. I was only gone at the maximum 45 minutes. God, how could I've been so stupid."

"Mr. Caldwell, don't worry. I'll have an all-points bulletin issued for the entire Rochester area in a few minutes. We'll find your father in plenty of time so he can get some rest before playing tomorrow. The story of you and your father is amazing. It means so much to those families that have parents suffering from Alzheimer's. We'll do everything we can in our power to find him," replied the officer.

"Thanks officer. I feel certain that you and your Police Department will do everything they can to find my father. Thank you again and I'll be waiting for a patrol car."

Mikey hung up the phone and walked back outside to wait for the police car.

About an hour earlier...

Charlie was sleeping lightly and heard the car start. He opened the door, and by the time he looked outside. Mikey was pulling out of the parking lot and heading down the road. Charlie was suddenly alone and desperate. "Mikey's going home. He forgot me. Oh, no, I'm going to have to get back to San Antonio by myself. Oh no... Oh no," Charlie cried out loud.

Mikey never looked back at the room and failed to see Charlie open the door to the motel room. Charlie watched as the car disappeared. He walked across the parking lot and out to the highway. He began walking in the direction of Charlie drove off to. As he walked across the first intersection, he was oblivious to the car approaching from the right. Charlie kept walking, not thinking about any danger of the car hitting him.

The driver of the car saw Charlie walking across the unmarked intersection and assumed that he was going to walk on and step up on the curb. He didn't think about Charlie stopping short of the curb for a short time. He stopped at the stop sign and began making his turn to the right when he heard a bump on the car and saw Charlie falling toward the curb. "Oh my God, I think I just hit this guy. Shit! That is all that I need." He thought to himself.

The driver got out of the car and walked around to Charlie who was just getting up. "Sir, I am very sorry. I thought that you were already on the curb. I am very sorry. Are you all right?" the driver asked.

"Yes," replied Charlie in a shaky voice.

"Sir, are you sure? If you want, I can take you to the hospital and so you can get checked out."

"No, I'm Okay," Charlie said. "I don't need to go to the hospital. I need to get home."

"Okay, tell you what, I will take you home. Where do you live?" asked the driver.

"I live in San Antonio," replied Charlie.

"San Antonio? San Antonio, Texas?" the man asked.

"Yes, I live in San Antonio, Texas."

"Sir, I can't take you all the way to San Antonio, Texas. If you were going to San Antonio tonight, how were you going to get there?" the man driving the car asked. "You are not planning to catch a ride there, are you?"

"Mikey is going to drive me to San Antonio, but I think he left early and forgot me."

"Well, I can take you to the interstate. If he's going to drive to San Antonio, your friend will have to drive by there. Maybe you can rest in the restaurant until he comes. If he doesn't show up, I am sure that you will be able to catch a ride in the morning. However, you have a long way to go," the driver added.

The driver drove the seven miles to the interstate and dropped Charlie off at the truck stop. Before Charlie got out of the car, the man asked, "Sir, are you sure that you are Okay? If you want, I can still take you by the hospital. Let them check you out just to make sure nothing is wrong."

Charlie didn't respond to the man but simply got out of the car and slowly walked toward the restaurant at the truck stop.

The driver of the car shook his head, and slowly drove off, not sure if he was doing the right thing.

Charlie walked in the restaurant at the truck stop and sat down in one of the booths by the window. He needed to be by the window so he could see Mikey when he drove up to pick him up.

The waitress walked up to Charlie and gave him a menu. "What can I get you to drink, sir?" She asked.

Charlie looked up at the waitress and said, "Mikey is going to pick me up."

"Okay Sir. Can I get you coffee while you wait," she asked.

"Yes, I would like a cup of coffee," Charlie replied.

The waitress brought Charlie his coffee and asked, "How about a piece of apple pie with the coffee?"

Charlie's eyes lit up. "Yes, I like apple pie," he responded.

The waitress quickly bought Charlie a slice of deep-dish apple pie. She placed it in the microwave for a few minutes to heat it up a bit so it was a bit warm. "Here you go sweetie," she said as she placed the slice of apple pie on the table.

Charlie didn't realize that it has been well over eight hours since he last ate anything and devoured the pie within a few bites. It was delicious. He then sipped his coffee as he waited for Mikey to come and pick him up.

The waitress filled and refilled Charlie's coffee cup several times during the next few hours. Finally she said, "Sir, we are getting ready to change shifts, and I need to close my register. Can you pay for the pie and coffee now?" She asked.

Charlie looked at her with a questioning look on his face. "Mikey will pay for it when he picks me up."

"We'll, it doesn't seem that your Mikey is coming," she said, somewhat upset with the free loader who took advantage of her. "The coffee and the pie are on me. You enjoy your evening, and I hope Mikey comes soon. If he doesn't show up in the next few minutes, you may have to wait outside," she added.

Charlie didn't look up, but kept staring at the window waiting for Mikey.

Meanwhile...

Two Rochester Police Department patrol cars arrived at the Best Western motel at the same time. A tall office got out of the first car and walked up to Mikey. "Sir, I'm Officer Barry Johnson, and we'll find your father. Let's go over the last time you saw him again."

"Okay, it was about seven forty-five this evening. My dad was asleep on the bed in room one-one-five and I needed to get him some clothes to wear tomorrow and other items to get us through the night. I left him and drove to Wal-Mart right down the road. I bought the stuff we needed and stopped by McDonalds on the way back. I was back at the room by eight-thirty at the latest. He was not in the room and the door was open. That was the last time I saw him," replied Mikey.

"Alright, we have issued an all-points bulletin for an elderly man wearing plastic rain pants with a light blue shirt. You can be assured that every police officer in this area will be looking for your father. If he is on the street, we will find him. Now, let's go over where you think he might be heading. Was there any indication of anything that you know of that might help us?" the officer asked.

"No, there's nothing I can think of. He did say several times today that he was ready to go home to San Antonio. I told him that we would be going back home real soon. You don't think that he was thinking about going back to San Antonio by himself, do you?" Mikey asked.

"Sir, a person with Alzheimer's may do anything. He may be walking down some side street at the moment thinking that he's only a few blocks from being home. You never know what a person with that condition may be doing or thinking. We have frequent reports of people with Alzheimer's missing and, so far, we have a perfect record in finding them," the officer said.

"Okay, and thanks for the help, Officer. I appreciate the effort you and your officers are making to safely find my father," replied Mikey.

"No problem, Sir. That's what we're here for. We'll go out and drive around the immediate area now. I suggest you wait in your room. If we find him, we'll bring him right back."

"Thank you again for your help," replied Mikey as he watched Officer Johnson get in the patrol car and drive away.

It was now one in the morning and Charlie was still sitting in the booth with his eyes glued on the parking lot. He really expected that Mikey would soon be picking him up and taking him home. The new waitresses were ignoring Charlie as the previous waitress told them that he was waiting for someone to come and pick him up. "Mikey is coming... Mikey is coming..." Charlie kept repeating to himself softly.

Officer Johnson drove by the Best Western and saw Mikey standing outside the door. He pulled the patrol car in and stopped near Mikey's room and rolled down the window.

Mikey walked up to the car and asked, "Do you have any news on my father?"

"Not yet, Mister Caldwell," replied Officer Johnson. "We have every patrol car available looking for him. We won't give up until we find him. Sir, we will find him. He's probably holed up somewhere and sleeping. When he wakes up and moves, we'll spot him for sure. Why don't you get some sleep? There's not a lot you can do and it would be best for you to be rested when we do find him."

With that news, Mikey reluctantly walked back to his room and lay down on top of the bed. He left the door ajar just in case Charlie found his way back.

It was now about an hour before the morning shift came on duty at the truck stop. The sun was about to break the horizon and Charlie was still looking at the parking lot. One waitress decided it was time to do something about the person occupying the booth the entire night. She walked up and Charlie didn't notice her. She tapped him on the shoulder and asked, "Sir, your friend doesn't look like he's going to show up. Can I call you a taxi?"

Charlie looked at her and said, "Okay, I can use a taxi to take me home."

The waitress called the local cab company and soon a taxi was waiting in front of the restaurant. The waitress again tapped Charlie on the shoulder and said, "Sir, your taxi is here."

"Okay," Charlie said as he got up and walked through the doors and outside. He stood there silently in front of the taxi, looking around. Finally, the taxi driver got out of the car and asked, "Are you the person that called for a cab?"

"Okay," Charlie said and opened the door to the cab and got in.

"Where will you be going this morning?" asked the cabby.

"I need to go to San Antonio," replied Charlie.

The taxi driver looked at Charlie in silence for a second before responding. "San Antonio... San Antonio, Texas. Sir, I can only take you someplace in the Rochester area. I cannot take you to San Antonio."

"Can you take me to Mikey?" Charlie asked.

"Who is Mikey and where is he at?" the driver asked back.

"Mikey is my caddie and he's probably waiting for me at the motel."

"Which motel is he at?" the driver asked.

"I don't know. We played golf and went to the motel. Mikey left me," Charlie said as he began to cry.

The taxi driver realized that he was not dealing with someone with a full deck and said, "Sir, let me see if I can find out some more information." He grabbed the microphone and called the main office. "Yeah, I have a pickup at the truck stop on Clover Street. The passenger seems to be confused and says he wants to go to San Antonio, Texas. He's now saying something about finding his caddie. What do you want me to do with this passenger?"

"Hold on a second, I believe there was a police report earlier this morning about looking out for an older person suffering from Alzheimer's. Yes, here it is. Is he wearing rain pants and a light blue shirt?"

"Yes, that is what he's wearing," replied the driver.

"Hold on and stay right there. I'll call the police department and they should be there in a few minutes to take over."

"Okay, I'll wait until the police come," replied the driver as he hung up the phone.

He got back out of the cab and told Charlie that someone was coming to help him. They should be there in a few moments. As they waited, the driver decided to strike up a conversation. "Sir, what is your name?" he asked.

"My name is Charlie."

"Hello Charlie, my name is Derek and I live in Rochester. I understand that you live in San Antonio, Texas."

"Yes, I live in San Antonio," replied Charlie.

"What brings you to Rochester?"

"I'm playing golf with my caddie. Mikey is my caddie."

"Playing golf, huh? Where are you playing?" the driver asked.

"I think we were playing on a golf course. I don't know the name. I can't remember things very well," Charlie said without emotion.

"No problem," replied the driver as he saw the police car turn into the parking lot.

The patrol car drove up just behind the taxi and the policeman got out and walked up to the taxi and opened the back door. "Hello Mister Caldwell, we've been looking for you all night. Are you alright?" he asked.

"I'm Okay. Where is Mikey? He was supposed to pick me up."

"I'll take you to Mikey right now. Let's get in my car and we'll be there in a couple of minutes. Mikey is waiting for you," replied the officer.

"Okay," said Charlie as he slid out of the back of the taxi and walked towards the open door of the patrol car.

As they drove back to the motel, the officer asked, "Mister Caldwell, I'll be rooting for you today. What time do you tee off?"

"I don't know," Charlie said. "I don't think I am playing golf today. I want to go home and see Diane."

"I think you are supposed to be playing golf and will be playing today with Tom Watson this afternoon in the final round. Aren't you excited?"

"I don't know Tom Watson. Does he play golf too?"

182

"You should know Tom Watson. He's a very famous golfer. Who did you play with yesterday?" the officer asked.

"I can't remember who it was. Mikey is my caddie and he knows who I played with. Ask Mikey," Charlie replied.

"Okay, well good luck today," replied the officer as he pulled into the parking lot of the motel near room 115. He was glad to see that Mikey was standing outside the motel room.

Mikey walked out and met the patrol car. He opened the door and his father slid out. Mikey, reached out and gave his dad a huge hug, "Dad, we have been looking for you all night. Where have you been?" Mikey asked.

"I was waiting for you to pick me up and take me home to San Antonio. You never came and I was worried. I want to go to sleep now. I am very sleepy."

Charlie walked past Mikey and into the room. He took his rain pants off and crawled into bed. He was fast asleep in minutes.

Mikey thanked the officer and followed his father into the room, closing the door behind him. He sat down in a chair and watched his father sleep before nodding off himself.

The two hadn't been asleep for very long when Mikey heard the commotion outside the motel room. Then, someone knocked on the door. Mikey opened the door and there were three news vans outside with reporters setting up their equipment. "Mister Caldwell, we understand your father was missing last night and you've just found him. Can we get an interview?" the reporter asked.

"No, please. My father is asleep and I want him to get his rest. Please be quiet and let him sleep. We'll give an interview after he wakes up. I expect to wake him up around noon. That should give us plenty of time to make it to the tournament before his tee time at 2:30pm. Please be quiet now."

There were other questions from several reporters but Mikey ignored them and walked back into the room, closing the door behind him. To his relief, everything was quiet outside.

Chapter Thirteen

Charlie woke up around eleven in the morning and staggered into the bathroom. He turned the light on and his image in the mirror caught his attention. "Who is this person staring back in the mirror?" he thought. He stopped dead in his tracks, just staring intently at the other person looking back at him. After a few moments that seemed like an eternity, Charlie came back to his limited senses and wondered why he was in the bathroom. "What was I doing?" he asked silently.

"Oh, yes, I got to pee!" he said with some excitement. He relieved himself and looked back in the mirror. "What else do I need to do?" he thought. He looked around the sink and saw several objects when he remembered the other thing he needed to do. I've got to brush my teeth and looked fervently for a toothbrush. "Where's my toothbrush?" he asked loudly.

The noise in the bathroom woke Mikey up and he quickly entered the bathroom to see his father scouring the small room, looking for a toothbrush. "Dad, I had to get you a new toothbrush and it is in the plastic bag on the sink. Here, let me open it for you," he said as he took the bag and retrieved the toothbrush. He then opened the plastic container and squeezed some toothpaste on the bristles and handed it to his father.

"There you go Dad. Now you can brush your teeth. Why don't you take a nice, warm shower too? I'll turn the water on for you." Mikey reached down and turned the shower on and then touched the water to make sure it wasn't too hot or too cold. "Dad, your shower is ready. When you finish brushing your teeth, take your shirt off and jump in the shower.

Meanwhile, I'll see if we can't get some breakfast delivered to the room."

Charlie didn't say anything or acknowledge what was just said. He was totally focused on the one task at hand, brushing his teeth. He finished and rinsed off his toothbrush. "Mikey," he called out. "Can I take a shower now?"

"Yes, Dad, I've already got the water going so take off your clothes and jump in the shower."

"Okay," replied Charlie, as he took his clothes off and stepped into the shower.

"Dad, don't forget to pull the curtain back so you don't get water all over everything," Mikey added.

Soon Charlie was in the shower, enjoying the feeling of the warm water flowing off his head and over his body. He liked the feeling of taking a shower.

Mikey opened the door and looked outside. The news vans were still there and when he opened the door, everyone scrambled to be the first to get a shot of him. "Dad is up now and taking a shower. Tell me, is there anyone here that will run down to McDonalds for us and get a couple of Egg McMuffins, two coffees and two orange juices?" Mikey asked to the reporters.

Nobody answered immediately and one voice from the back said, "Sure, I'll do that for you. Do you want cream and sugar for the coffee?" the person asked.

"No, black is fine and thank you," replied Mikey.

At that time, the questions from all the other reporters came on fast and furiously.

"No questions now. Thank you all, but we need to get ready. We'll see you at the course," replied Mikey as he closed the door.

Charlie was still in the shower when the knock came at the door. Mikey opened the door and it was the reporter delivering the McDonald's order. "Mister Caldwell, here is your order," he said as he handed the bag to Mikey.

"Thank you very much. I tell you what, meet me and my father at the driving range today in about an hour and we'll give you an exclusive ten-minute interview. The questions need to be directed at me and not my father. He really can't answer your questions and I don't want anybody making fun of his condition," Mikey said.

Mikey turned toward the other reporters and added, "The interview on the driving range will be with this reporter only and not the rest of you. He was the one that took the initiative and went to McDonalds for us. Sorry, but maybe you should have stepped up earlier," Mikey said with a little pride in his voice.

Mikey closed the door and went to the bathroom where his father was still standing under the shower. "Dad, we have breakfast ready. Why don't you get out of the shower, dry off and put these new clothes on. I'll have your Egg McMuffin, coffee and orange juice ready for you."

"Okay," said Charlie. "I'm hungry."

He was soon dressed and walked into the room and sat down at the table. Mikey had the television on and was watching the local news channel where the big story was the event with Charlie last night. It seems that the taxi driver or the taxi cab company leaked the story to the news early this morning. It was now the biggest news story on television.

Charlie was quickly devouring his sandwich when he saw his picture on the television. "Mikey, look at the TV, I'm on television, playing golf. I like playing golf."

The accompanying story meant nothing to him and he quickly turned his attention back to the food in front of him.

However, Mikey was interested in the story and watched intensely. They interviewed several of the other senior tour players, asking them what they thought about a person with severe Alzheimer's playing a tour event. Without exception, the players thought that having a disease like Alzheimer's should not necessarily keep you from playing a tour event as long as it didn't disrupt the play of others. However, there were some golfers that thought Charlie was provided exceptions to the rules and this was unfair to the other competitors.

The final interview was with Tom Watson and he was extremely supportive of Charlie and his playing in the Senior Open. "Charlie and Jay were directly ahead of us yesterday and I watched his play on most of the holes. Jay Haas said it was really enjoyable playing the Charlie. I'll tell you one thing; according to Jay, Charlie can really hit the ball. His caddie would hand him a club and tell him where to hit it and the next thing you know, the ball was flying toward the hole. "

The reporter then asked Watson, "But wouldn't you find it a bit disturbing if he kept asking you your name? We asked that same question to Jay Haas earlier. We counted the times that he asked Jay about his name but also wanted to know if he also played golf. I believe he asked the same question 8 times during the round. In an interview yesterday, Jay said that it was a bit disturbing?"

"I spoke with Jay last night and he said it was not disturbing at all. I have friends who are suffering from the onset of this disease and there are many, many other families that watch their parents, or loved ones just deteriorate in front of their eyes. Having Charlie asking me my name several times will be nothing. I will consider it an honor to be able to tell him my name," replied Watson. "However, I am thinking about wearing a name tag today," he added, laughing and smiling.

The interview with Watson made Mikey smile. When he first met Watson on the driving range the first day of the tournament, Mikey could tell that Watson was an outstanding gentleman. He was glad that it ended up that Charlie and Watson would be playing together on the last day.

Charlie finished his Egg McMuffin and orange juice. He was up and back in the bathroom, brushing his hair. Mikey was already dressed and ready to go when Charlie walked out of the bathroom.

"I'm ready to go home Mikey," he said.

"No Dad, we're going to play golf one more day. You get to play with Tom Watson again. You remember him, don't you?"

"I don't want to play golf today. I want to go home. Let's go home," Charlie said.

"Dad, let's make a deal. We'll play golf today and we'll try to get Watson to make a bet for hamburgers after the round. That way, you can win us a couple of hamburgers that we can eat on the way home. How does that sound?" asked Mikey.

"Bet for hamburgers? Okay, we can get a big hamburger before we fly home to San Antonio," Charlie replied with excitement in his voice. "Hamburgers... we're going to be playing golf for hamburgers."

Mikey put the toiletries and Charlie's old clothes in the Wal-Mart bag and the two opened the door and walked through the reporters. There were dozens of questions and each reporter was trying to get the picture of the day.

"Charlie, where did you go last night?" one asked.

"Mister Caldwell, were you really lost?" asked another.

"Gentlemen, please. Let us get through. We need to go to the course, please," Mikey yelled out. They finally got to the car and had to wait for one of the vans to move before they could back out. Mikey locked the doors so they couldn't get in as Charlie was simply looking around at all the commotion.

"Mikey, what are all the people here for? What do they want?" he asked.

"Dad, these are reporters and they want to know who is going to win the hamburger bet today."

"Oh yes, we are going to win a hamburger today," Charlie said, again with lots of excitement.

Soon, the two were driving onto the grounds of Oakhill Country Club in Richmond. They drove up to the gate and the guard looked at the pass on the front windshield and looked in the car. "Oh, hello Mister Caldwell, it's good to see you today. Good luck out there."

Charlie looked at the gate guard and simply said, "Okay."

Mikey drove the car up to valet parking and the two got out. He gave the car-keys to one of the attendants and the two walked into the player's locker room. The locker room talk must have been centered on Charlie as everything suddenly quieted when they two walked into the room.

Tom Watson was the first to speak. "Hey Charlie, I heard you had an exciting night. I'm glad to see that everything turned out well and you're here. Are you ready to play some golf today?"

"Hi… I'm sorry, I can't remember your name but I know your face, I think," replied Charlie.

"My name is Tom. It's Okay if you can't remember it. I'll see you on the tee box," Watson said as he turned toward the locker room door.

"Okay, Mikey says that I'm playing you for a hamburger bet today," Charlie said, laughing quietly.

"Okay, a hamburger bet it is," said Watson. "I love playing golf for a hamburger," he added as he walked out of the player's locker room.

Other golfers said hello to Charlie and some talked briefly about his golf game. You could tell by the conversations that most admired the golfing skill he demonstrated in the first three days of the tournament.

Bernard Langer was due to play in the group just in front and he gently touched Charlie on the shoulder and said, "Charlie, go out there and win a hamburger from Tom."

Charlie looked up at Langer and smiled, saying, "Okay."

Mikey helped Charlie put on his one pair of golf shoes and the two headed toward the practice range. The reporters were there in force and some were in the middle of interviewing other golfers when they saw Mikey and Charlie walk up. Most of the reporters quickly ended their interview to get a few words from the story of the day.

Mikey looked around and found the reporter that got them the breakfast this morning. "Hello," he said pointing to the person. "Bring your camera and come on up." Mikey lifted the rope and asked them to come through, which they did.

They went to one side of the driving range and away from the others. Mikey handed Charlie a pitching wedge and said, "Dad, you go ahead and hit some balls while I talk with these folks. They're the ones that brought us breakfast this morning."

Charlie looked up at the camera crew and said, "Okay."

Mikey began the interview with some rules. They were not supposed to direct any questions to Charlie and Mikey would try to answer all of their questions. The interview would need to stop in ten minutes, too.

The first question was really not a question as the reporter summed up the events that led up to today. "Sir, your father entered the US Senior Open qualification tournament and played in San Antonio. We understand that the PGA questioned his inability to recall and record his scores for the day and disqualified him. However, due to the overwhelming response from the public, they changed their ruling and gave him an exemption. Is that correct?"

"Yes, that is fairly accurate. Dad was asked to verify a score he made on one of the holes and he said he didn't remember.

He wasn't able to remember what he had on that hole. According to Rule Six, the golfer must be responsible for recording his scores. I kept the score for him but wasn't available when they began reviewing the scores after the round. The official that was recording the score had a question about one of the holes. He asked dad what he made on the hole and dad said I can't remember. Since dad could not remember his score, the USGA had to disqualify him under the rules. Later on, they reviewed the rule and determined that dad did not attempt to gain an advantage and therefore his score should be counted. Since they already announced the actual qualifiers, they then determined to offer dad an exemption."

"How long has your father been playing golf?" the reporter asked.

"My father started playing golf when he was in high school. He played in college for the University of Houston and then turned professional. He played in a few professional events after college but decided that he really wasn't cut out to play on the tour. He has been the head professional for Pecan Valley Country Club in San Antonio, Texas for almost thirty years."

"Do you play golf, too?" the reporter asked.

"I've played golf growing up but I cannot compete with my father."

"Mister Caldwell, can we discuss Charlie and how he's coping with Alzheimer's?" the reporter asked.

"Sure you can. My father and I do not have any secrets concerning this disease. However, please do not ask him if he has the disease. My father sincerely believes he simply has memory problems like many other older people. As many of you know, Alzheimer's is a disease that affects thousands of Americans each year and it can be very trying on the family. Fortunately, we discovered that my father happened to still have the basics of a good golf swing in his body. This does not require good short-term memory and, as you can see, he's played golf pretty well in the last few days."

"Yes, he is playing extremely well. When did he first suspect that he was having memory problems?" the reporter asked.

"Well, I believe he began to worry about it a couple of years ago. It started out with him forgetting some minor things at home and at work. He had trouble remembering names of club members at Pecan Valley Country Club in San Antonio and then other issues happened. This really worried him but he tried to keep it to himself. The owners of Pecan Valley are very supportive of dad and gave him an excellent retirement package. He is still a frequent fixture around the club."

"Alright, Mister Caldwell, my last question is do you think your father can hold it together today and win the US Senior Open?"

"Dad can only go out and play one shot at a time. He has no control over how well the other golfers play. These guys are really good, too. I will say that dad thinks he's playing for a hamburger bet with Tom Watson, so he'll be as focused as he can be," Mikey said.

As he was turning to join his father on the range, Mikey stopped and said to the reporter, "Thank you for the breakfast this morning and thank you for making this interview very enjoyable for both of us."

"Mister Caldwell, thank you and we will be following you the entire round. Best of luck to you and your dad," he added.

"Thanks and we'll be watching for you on the course," Mikey said.

Mikey then turned his attention to his father and watched him hit the five iron straight as an arrow, each ball landed in a tight pattern about 180 yards away. "Dad, that looks real smooth. How do you feel?"

"Okay," replied Charlie.

Mikey took the five-iron from his father and handed him the now famous five- wood. "Let's hit a few off the deck," Mikey said.

Charlie replied with the usual, "Okay."

Mikey watch his dad take the club and single out a ball and move it to a clean spot of grass. Charlie took the club back with a smooth, one-motion and momentarily stopped at the top. He then began the down swing slowly and increasing club head speed until after contacting the ball. The ball headed off toward the target line, rising, and then slowly arching back toward the earth. It landed about 210 yards away and bounced forward.

The next club was Charlie's three-wood and, with the same smooth swing, he launched the ball toward the two hundred and fifty yard sign. The ball bounced and hit the sign squarely.

There was a large gallery of fans behind the practice area and most were focused on watching Charlie hit shots. Someone in the group shouted out, "Charlie, bet you can't hit that sign again."

Mikey and Charlie both looked back at the crowd and were amazed at the size of the gallery. Only a handful of people were watching any of the other professionals as they went through their routines. Charlie looked at the crowd and waved.

This caused a bit of laughter from a few in the gallery and lots of chatter.

Charlie used the club and dragged another ball to a smooth patch of grass. It was a repeat of the same, smooth swing. The ball lifted off the ground with a bit higher arch. This time the ball hit the sign directly, without bouncing. Charlie laughed out loud but his laughter couldn't be heard from the loud applause the gallery gave him. Mikey was worried of the commotion upsetting the other professionals using the range, but when he looked, the only other golfer on the range was Tom Watson. Tom was also clapping.

Charlie looked back at the crowd and again waved.

After hitting the driver and then a few additional wedges, Mikey told Charlie that they should stop hitting balls and get something to eat before putting a bit. "Dad, let's grab a sandwich before we go out. What do you say?"

"Okay," replied Charlie.

"Charlie, can I get your autograph?" one of the fans shouted out.

Mikey started to decline but Charlie was already walking their way. He was happy when the fans began holding their programs, caps and other things for him to sign. He took the first cap from one of the fans and signed "Charlie," before handing it back. He would have continued signing but Mikey intervened and told the fans that they needed to get ready for the round. "Charlie will be available to sign items later. We've got to get a bite before we play. Please excuse us," Mikey said.

He then grabbed Charlie's hand and shouldered the golf bag before heading off to the professional's dining area. The two went in and grabbed a couple of sandwiches and sat down at one of the tables. Charlie opened the can of Coke in front of him and took a short sip.

They were both focused on their sandwich and didn't notice the other golfer that joined them. "Gentlemen, do you mind if I join you?" he asked.

Mikey looked up and realized that it was Gary Player. He started to say sure but Charlie beat him to the punch and said, "Okay."

Player sat down and said, "Charlie, good luck today. I see you're playing with Tom Watson. Tom is a really nice man and one of the very best golfers we have on the Senior Tour."

Charlie just smiled.

"Good luck with the round today," Gary added.

Charlie looked at Gary Player and asked, "Do you play golf too?"

"Well, I try," replied Player. "However, I'm not playing as well as you. My group went out early and we just finished."

"What is your name," Charlie asked.

"Oh, I should have introduced myself. My name is Gary Player and I come from South Africa. Have you ever been to South Africa, Charlie?"

"No, I live in San Antonio, Texas. Mikey is going to take me home after we play golf."

"San Antonio is a beautiful city for sure," replied Player before Mikey cut him off.

"Excuse me, Mister Player, we need to go and putt a few balls before our tee time.

"Certainly, I understand. Good luck to you both. I'll be rooting for you."

"Thank you," replied Mikey. "Dad, let's go the bathroom before putting. We don't want to have the same accident as yesterday, do we?"

"What happened yesterday?" asked Charlie.

Mikey realized that there was no need for an explanation. "Nothing really happened," he replied as he escorted his father into the bathroom.

Soon, Charlie did everything he had to in the bathroom and was ready to go.

Mikey said, "Let's go and putt a few balls now. We tee off in 20 minutes."

"Okay," replied Charlie.

The two went out to the large, practice putting green and Mikey took three new balls out of the bag and placed them on the green. Charlie took the putter from Mikey and casually walked up and putted all three balls directly into the hole about five feet away.

The gallery had been watching Tom Watson putt but after Charlie sunk the first three putts, all eyes were now focused away from Tom.

After five or six minutes of putting, Mikey knew his dad was ready.

They walked through a large crowd to the number one tee box at Oak Hill Country Club.

Bernard Langer and Fred Couples had just teed off and were walking down the fairway when Charlie and Mikey walked up to the tee box. Soon, they were joined by Tom Watson and his caddie.

Tom walked up to Charlie and held out his hand. "Good luck, Charlie," he said.

Charlie shook Watson's hand and replied with, "Okay."

Watson smiled and added, "Don't forget, we're playing for a hamburger."

Charlie had a huge smile on his face and again replied, "Okay."

Watson just smiled and walked away to say a few words to the starter.

After a few minutes and the previous two golfers clearing the way, the starter said over the loudspeaker, "Ladies and Gentlemen. We now have the final group of the day. From Kansas City, Missouri, The winner of last year's Senior Open, Tom Watson."

The large gallery around the first tee erupted in a loud applause.

Watson acknowledged the applause and smiled at the crowd. He then gently placed a ball on the tee and went through his usual pre-swing routine. Watson hit his drive with pure perfection. It flew just past the point where the fair way drops down. The ball landed at the 260 yard mark and then bounced down the fairway another 30 or 40 yards.

The starter then announced the next golfer, "From San Antonio, Texas, Charlie Caldwell."

The gallery's applause seemed to be even greater than that for Tom Watson.

Unlike Tom Watson, Charlie simply walked up to the tee box, reached down and teed up an almost new Titleist golf ball.

Mikey walked up and told his father, "Hit in right at the middle of the fairway."

"Okay," replied Charlie. He looked down the fairway and then looked at the crowd and smiled. Just like on the driving range, he was smooth in the take away in the downswing was flawless. The ball went on almost the same flight path as Tom Watson's ball. As they walked down the fairway an enormous crowd followed them on both sides of the ropes. Charlie was walking with Tom Watson, and Tom was talking to Charlie all the way.

Mikey saw this and was wondering if Watson was trying to psych out Charlie. Then he thought to himself, "Charlie has got to be impossible to psych out." Nevertheless, he needed to separate Charlie, so he could prepare him for the next shot. The two balls were almost side to side, but Charlie's was a bit outside and would be the first to hit. It was 115 yards to the flag and Mikey handed Charlie a pitching wedge. The hole was slightly uphill, and there was a light wind blowing against them. Charlie took the same smooth swing as usual, and the ball took a flight directly at the pin. As soon as the ball left the club, Mikey knew that it would be short. The ball landed just short of the green and into the face of a steep bunker. Charlie looked at Mikey with a questioning look. "Mikey, that was too short, I think."

Mikey saw the disappointment in Charlie's face. "That was my fault, Dad. You hit the perfect shot and I under clubbed you. I'll make sure it doesn't happen again. You're playing very well and I can taste that hamburger already, how about you?"

"You bet, son. That hamburger is going to taste so good. Let's play golf," Charlie replied.

Mikey was shocked. This was the very first time in months that Charlie called Mikey 'son.' He thought to himself that this was the most in tuned he had seen his father in months. He actually carried on a conversation with another person and he knew I was his son and not his caddie.

Meanwhile, Tom Watson, being the pro that he is, noticed which club Mikey handed Charlie. He watched the shot, and based upon the results of Charlie's shot, Tom grabbed a nine iron. He took the same swing as Charlie and his ball was on a lower trajectory. It landed ten feet from the flag took a bounce and stopped just short of the hole.

The crowd applauded with enthusiasm as this was the Tom Watson they all knew. Charlie rarely made comments about another golfer's shot. However, at this time he made an exception. "That was a very nice shot, Tom" he said.

"Thanks Charlie. You had a good shot too, but it just came up a bit short. Keep your swing going and think positive. You will find your distance soon."

When they reached the sand trap and Mikey and Charlie both saw the predicament that they were in a golf ball was underneath the lip of the bunker and there appeared to be no way Charlie would be able to get it up and over the lip. Charlie looked at the shot and was perplexed. "Mikey," he said, "I don't have a good shot here. I may be able to get it over the lip of the trap but I will not be able to get it on the green. What do you think I should do?"

"Dad, I think the best thing would be to take an unplayable lie and drop it in the bunker. Knock it up on the green and take one putt for a bogey."

Charlie looked the shot over again and said, "I can get it over the lip of the bunker. I need a sand wedge," Charlie said, with his words making more and more sense to Mikey. He was still amazed at his father and how his conversations seemed to be perfectly normal.

Mikey handed his father a sand wedge and stood back out of the way.

Charlie walked around to the front of the bunker holding a sand wedge in hand and climbed up the steep face. He planted his right foot deep in the sand to give himself a firm footing. He took a huge backswing and accelerated down through the ball exploding a huge volume of sand toward the green. The ball caught the edge of the bunker, reflecting it straight up. It looked like it almost touched Charlie's right arm but Charlie knew it did touch him. So light was the touch that Mikey thought it was a clean hit. After barely touching Charlie the ball went straight up and came back down in the bunker, rolling backwards to a flat area.

Tom Watson also saw the shot from a different angle and he couldn't tell if the ball touched Charlie. He assumed the Charlie would be lying three in the bunker.

Mikey saw the shot and the result of the shot. "Dad, that's Okay. You're still laying three and can get on the green and make bogey."

"No Mikey, that ball touched me. You may not have seen it but it barely touched my arm on the way up. It did touch me and I have to take a penalty stroke."

"Dad, are you sure? To me it looked like the ball came very close but I could not tell if it touched you. It certainly didn't look like it touched you."

"Mikey, the ball did touch me. So let's go and play golf," Charlie said with anger in his voice.

Charlie took the same sand wedge and walked back out of the trap and knocked the sand from his shoes. He then looked at the situation and reentered the trap. He set up on the ball, dug his shoes in and quickly hit a sand shot that was too hard. The ball flew well over the green.

As he walked out of the trap he said to Mikey, "Son, we still have some golf to play on this hole."

Mikey raked the trap real quickly, grabbed the bag and hurried over to where Charlie was standing over his ball.

Meanwhile, Tom Watson was standing on the green away from the shots watching his opponent throw away shots. He had a sad look on his face as he liked Charlie. Watson is one of the many golfers on tour that pride themselves in winning tournaments and not because another golfer played poorly. However, the rules of golf are very strict and Tom knew he could do very little to help Charlie. Nevertheless, it was a bit sad.

Charlie looked his shot over very carefully. The ball was sitting down, deep in the rough. This would be as difficult as the second bunker shot. Charlie took the sand wedge, opened the blade and took a huge swing. The ball flew high and landed softly about ten feet from the pin. Charlie walked up to the ball on the green and took out a coin and marked the ball. He handed the ball to Mikey and looked at the line of the putt. Mikey cleaned the ball and handed it back to Charlie, who placed it very carefully in front of the mark. He then putted and watched as the ball curled around and stopped just outside of the hole. Charlie tapped it in and reached down to pick the ball out of the hole. There was a light applause, which Charlie acknowledged with a small smile.

Watson then walked up, placed his ball down on the mark and made the short putt for birdie three. Charlie ended up with a nine.

Charlie began the hole with a four shot lead over Tom Watson and a five shot lead over Bernard Langer. After the first hole, Charlie was now two behind Watson and one behind Langer, who also birdied the first hole.

The second hole at Oak Hill is a fairly simple par four with not a lot of trouble. Watson was first to hit and elected a three wood off the tee. It ended up in the center of fairway about 150 yards from the green. Charlie elected to go with the driver and hit a longer ball but was in the short rough.

Watson knocked his second ball on the green, about 20 feet from the pin. Charlie was about 115 yards from the green and reached out for Mikey to hand him a club. Mikey hesitated but picked the wedge again. "Dad, this is a wedge so hit it solid."

"Okay," replied Charlie.

Charlie hit a solid shot that flew directly over the pin. The ball took a short bounce and backed up to five feet from the pin.

The crowd erupted into a large applause and Charlie simply smiled back.

Watson was first to putt and almost made it two birdies in a row. Unlike the first hole, Charlie placed his ball down on the mark, stood up quickly and moved to the edge of the green. He appeared to be waiting for Tom to finish.

Mikey walked up to his father and whispered, "Dad, it's your putt."

Charlie responded, "Okay," and walked up to his ball. He quickly putted the ball without taking a good look at the hole. The ball went straight and true, dropping in the hole for a birdie three.

"Nice putt, Charlie," said Watson.

"Okay," Charlie replied with a barely visible smile on his face.

Mikey was the first to notice that the person he saw earlier on the first hole had left and the regular Charlie without his memory had returned. With the suddenness of just a few minutes, Charlie suddenly reverted back into the person with Alzheimer's.

Watson birdied another hole and ended up on the front at six under par for the tournament, while Charlie carded two birdies after taking a nine on the first hole and was at five under. Langer was even with Charlie before going into the back side.

Watson was leading the group as they transitioned between the ninth green and the tenth tee box. The roped off corridor was narrow and fans cheered loudly as the golfers walked by.

Many held their hands out, signaling for a 'high-five'. Watson just smiled at everyone and walked through without hitting any hands. Charlie was just in front of Mikey and he was trying to give everyone a 'high-five'.

Fans would shout out words of encouragement such as, "Go get-um Charlie," and "Charlie, you're the man!" Charlie replied to all with a simple "Okay."

The final group was finally on the tenth tee and Charlie was up first. "Dad, you're up," Mikey said.

"Okay," replied Charlie as he stood there in silence, not moving. He had a perplexed look on his face and Mikey realized that Charlie had forgotten where he was and what he was doing.

"Dad, you're going to play some golf with Tom Watson. You are hitting the ball first," Mikey said.

Charlie looked at Mikey with a lost look and replied, "Okay." He still didn't make a movement to tee his ball.

"Now what?" Mikey said to himself. Mikey was getting a bit nervous as he knew there was a time limit of five minutes between shots. "Dad, you've got to hit the golf ball. Please tee it up," he said anxiously.

"Mikey, I really don't want to play any more golf. Can we go home?" Charlie asked.

"We will go home after we play nine more holes. We have to finish the round."

"I don't want to finish," Charlie yelled quite loudly.

He threw the ball and tee down to the ground and stared angrily at Mikey.

The fans around the tee were absolutely stunned. It was totally quiet and you could actually hear a pin drop.

Mikey looked at Charlie with a perplexed look on his face, not really knowing what to do in this situation.

Tom saw this and decided to step in. He walked up to Charlie and whispered in his ear.

Charlie replied, "Okay," and proceeded to tee his ball up.

Mikey handed Charlie the driver and Charlie went straight to the ball and without a practice swing, laced a 265 yard drive straight down the middle of the fairway. Tom followed and again almost placed his ball on top of the ball already in the fairway.

"Nice drive, Charlie," Tom said as he walked off the tee box.

Mikey quickly caught up with the two golfers and asked Tom, "What did you whisper in my father's ear?"

"Oh, not much," Tom replied smiling broadly. "I just told Charlie that you would buy both of us a hamburger when we finished the round."

"Thanks, I was beginning to think that we would be leaving sooner than expected," Mikey said.

Tom and Charlie continued to walk down the fairway together.

"You know, Charlie. That hamburger is sure going to be good, huh?" Tom said.

"That hamburger will really taste good. Mikey is going to buy us both a hamburger."

Charlie was first to hit off the fairway. He was about 290 yards from the green and it was a very tight landing area for a three wood. Mikey handed Charlie a five iron and said, "Dad, let's go with a five iron. It will put us about 120 yards from the pin. Aim down the middle of the fairway."

Charlie took the five-iron and addressed the ball. He stopped his routine and looked at Tom. "What would you hit from here?" he asked.

Tom was shocked. He knew that even though it was inadvertent, Charlie had just committed a rules violation and it would cost him two shots. "Charlie, I can't tell you that. Just hit the ball," he said quickly.

Tom was now stuck in an unusual predicament. Charlie asked what club he would hit and that constituted asking for advice from someone other than your caddie. If he reported the violation, it would appear that he was calling Charlie on a rule violation just to have the two shots assessed to Charlie's score. If he didn't say anything, he could be held in violation for not reporting a known infraction of the rules.

Meanwhile, Charlie hit a perfect five-iron and was now lying in the middle of the fairway about one hundred and ten yards from the green.

Mikey heard his dad ask Tom what club he would hit from this spot and immediately realized that his dad violated a rule and must be assessed a two-shot penalty. He also saw Tom wince when he heard Charlie. Mikey waited until Tom hit a four iron to the center of the fairway, just a few yards in front of Charlie's ball. "Mr. Watson," he said, "I heard Charlie ask you what club you would hit and I think it is a violation of the rule. Please add a two shot penalty to his score on this hole."

Tom looked at Mikey and was relieved that the burden of reporting the violation was removed from his shoulder. "Mikey, I will do this but will also have the rules committee review the calling. Charlie already had the club you gave him in his hand and was set up to hit the shot. I don't believe that he was asking me what club I would hit as advice. I think he was just trying to make conversation," Tom responded.

As the group was walking toward their balls, Tom motioned for the rules committee person to come over. Mikey watched as Tom related what happened and he overheard Tom saying that he wasn't really asking the question for advice but simply making conversation. The rules committee person then went to the side of the fairway and used his wireless to contact the main committee.

Charlie was the first to hit and Mikey handed him a pitching wedge. Charlie never looked at the club to verify which club he was hitting, but simply took a short practice swing before hitting a beautiful shot that hit five feet from the pin, took one short bounce and stopped right by the hole.

The crowd on the ropes and around the green again erupted into a loud roar. As usual, Charlie just smiled at the crowd.

Tom followed with another shot that hit beyond the pin and caught the down-slope, eventually stopping some forty-five feet from the pin. A few people clapped, but it was nothing like the response when Charlie hit his shot.

Charlie marked his ball and stepped back to allow Tom to putt. Tom's putt came up short of the hole and needed to make a five footer to save par. He missed this putt and tapped in for a bogey.

Charlie tapped his putt in and the group noticed one of the officials was standing by the edge of the green. He confirmed that the main rules committee heard what happened and made the ruling that it was indeed a violation of the rule. There was nothing in the rule book that indicated it wasn't a violation if the person didn't intend to use the information to his advantage. It was simply a violation of the rule which stated that one golfer cannot ask for club selection or any other advice that would enable him to make a club selection. Therefore, Charlie would be assessed a two-shot penalty and both players would record a six on the par-five tenth hole.

The crowd around the green applauded feverishly when Charlie tapped in for what they all thought was an easy birdie. When the score was posted on the scoreboard, the applause turned in a low, muffled roar. They had no idea of the penalty that was just assessed.

Both players in the last group matched par through the fourteenth hole and walked up in time to see Bernard Langer make a birdie on the short par-three seventeenth. The crowd again erupted and Mikey looked at the scoreboard. Langer was the leader and one shot ahead of Tom and two ahead of Charlie.

Charlie was first to hit and Mikey looked at the pin sheet to determine the exact distance to the hole before handing Charlie a six-iron. Again, Charlie never looked at the club but simply took his short practice swing and then hit a high shot that flew directly over the pin and stopped about fifteen feet away.

The crowd again exploded into applause and some ignored the warning from the officials to not allow groups of people to shout out one golfer's name in unison. A handful began shouting "Charlie, Charlie." This reaction caused other fans to also begin the same chant. The marshals had to quiet the crowd and were running around trying to silence them. After what seemed like minutes, the crowd silenced enough to allow Tom to hit. His shot came up short of the green and rolled backwards, finally stopping in a swell well below the green.

Some fans got word from the news media of the ruling back on number ten and thought that Tom called the penalty on Charlie. They did not understand the situation and the fact that Tom was actually in favor of Charlie not being penalized. Some of these fans clapped and some even booed Tom's shot.

Mikey observed this and as he walked by Tom, he apologized for the situation. "That's alright, Mikey. These are our fans and I can certainly understand what they are feeling. Hell, I'm feeling the same way myself."

As Mikey walked on toward the green, Tom added, "Mikey, you're a great caddie and an even better son. Thanks."

Mikey smiled as he hurried to catch his father who was well ahead, walking by the ropes and slapping hands.

Charlie marked his ball and watched Tom walk up to the green and then back down to his ball. He retrieved a sand-wedge and hit a beautiful chip that followed the slope of the hill and landed on the front of the green. It began a long roll toward the hole.

Mikey watched the ball and immediately knew it was going to be close, real close. The ball continued up the green and rolled up to the edge of the hole, stopping momentarily before falling in. Everyone in the crowd clapped, some even yelled. Despite their feelings of what happened on ten, they all appreciated seeing a great shot from a great golfer. Even Charlie clapped when the ball finally dropped in the hole.

Tom walked up the slope, smiled and even took off his visor as he waved to the crowd. He picked the ball out of the hole to another ovation.

Everything quieted quickly when Charlie took his putter and made a quick look at the line. He placed the ball down and put the marker in his pocket. Like every other stroke this week, Charlie took one practice swing and placed the putter behind the ball. In one smooth motion he sent the ball rolling toward and directly into the hole.

The noise from the crowd was now deafening. Now, many ignored the unofficial ban of chanting "Charlie" and more and more took up the chant in unison. The USGA thought the chant was not in the best interest of the tournament and asked that it not be done today. Their ban on the chant worked for 17 holes but was now totally ignored. It now seemed as if every person on the golf course was yelling "Charlie…Charlie."

Charlie was showing a broad smile and again slapped hands with the crowd as they walked to the eighteenth tee box.

With two holes left to play, Bernard Langer was tied with Tom Watson at five under while Charlie was third at four under. Langer made a bogey on the seventeenth to fall one behind Watson and even with Charlie.

Tom and Charlie both hit great drives on the long, par-four finishing hole at Oak Hill Country Club. Charlie had two hundred and twenty yards to the pin, while Watson was near the two hundred yard marker. They arrived at their ball about the time they heard the roar from the crowd reacting to Langer making a long putt for a birdie. He was now again tied with Tom Watson and one ahead of Charlie.

Mikey looked at his father who was really showing signs of being tired now. "Dad, this is our last hole so let's win us a couple of hamburgers. Okay?" he asked.

"Okay, I like hamburgers," replied Charlie.

Mikey selected the three-wood and said, "Hit it in the center of the green."

"Okay," replied Charlie as he took the three-wood from Mikey. He took the standard practice swing before unleashing a powerful stroke that sent the ball flying towards the green. It came in a bit low and straight as an arrow. It landed in front of the green, bounced once and began the long roll toward the back of the green. The ball kept rolling and rolling on the long green before finally stopping about 15 feet short of the pin. The entire gallery was now forty or fifty deep around the green, watching from balconies or anywhere where they could get a view of history being made. In unison, they continued chanting Charlie's name like never-ending thunder.

Charlie heard the applause and the chanting that followed. He turned toward Mikey and said, "Do you hear that, Mikey? Everyone's calling out my name. What do you think they want?"

"Dad, they're just happy to see you play golf. The only thing they want is for you to make the putt. Make this putt and we'll be in a playoff," replied Mikey.

"What is a playoff?" asked Charlie.

The crowd was still chanting, "Charlie… Charlie," and only slightly quieted so Tom could hit his shot.

As he was getting ready, Charlie and Mikey quietly continued their conversation. "If you make the putt, you will be tied for first place with Bernard Langer and Tom Watson. That means that we'll have to play a few more holes to beat them both. That's what a playoff is."

"Okay," replied Charlie.

They both watched Tom hit a shot that matched Charlie's. It had the same, low trajectory and landed just short of the green. It ended up just past the hole, leaving a short but tricky downhill putt for birdie.

As they were walking toward the green, Charlie turned toward Mikey and said, "You told me that I only had to play one round of golf today, Mikey. I don't want to play any more golf today. I am going home after we finish this hole. Do you understand?"

Mikey realized that the sudden change in plans pissed his father off and out jumped the more normal Charlie Caldwell. "Dad, you need to play so we can win a hamburger."

"I don't want a hamburger anymore," replied Charlie, sounding very angry.

As they continued walking toward the green and the loud applause, Mikey realized that having his father play professional golf was not necessarily for Charlie, nor was it for Mikey. Charlie was actually playing for all of the golfers and non-golfers that somehow discovered they had this terrible disease. Mikey wanted his father to have fun but he also wanted the fans to enjoy themselves too.

Mikey reached out his hand and his father reacted by holding his son's hand as they walked toward the green. Saying in a loud voice and turning toward his father, Mikey added, "Dad, I love you. Knock this putt close and we'll go home."

"Okay," replied Charlie.

Tom Watson was first to putt and took his time lining everything up. He needed this putt to win outright by one shot over Langer and one shot over Charlie should he make birdie. The tricky downhill putt was his masterpiece but he knew immediately that his stroke was a bit timid and the ball stopped inches short of the hole. He tapped in for par and was tied with Bernard Langer. There would certainly be a playoff this afternoon. The only question now would be two or three golfers.

Charlie took the putter from Mikey and replaced his ball, this time tossing his marker to the side. His normal routine was to take a short practice swing, then step up to the ball. This time, he took three practice swings before stepping up to the ball. Instead of the stroke being smooth, it was a bit quick. The ball took off toward the hole and began to slow down as it neared the hole. It was angling right but to everyone, it still looked like it would be another great putt. The slope of the green took it and it slid by the hole and stopped a few inches away.

The crowd thought it was going in and began their chant, 'Charlie… Charlie,' when the ball left the putter. As it slid by the hole, the chants and claps turned into a dull, "Auhhhhhhhh" sound.

Charlie tapped in for his par and turned toward Mikey. He was handing Mikey the putter but Mikey dropped the putter on the ground and hugged his father. The crowd was now back to chanting "Charlie… Charlie."

As he hugged his father, Mikey said, "Dad, let's go home."

"Okay," replied Charlie.

Tom Watson walked over and stuck out his hand to Charlie.

Charlie started to take the hand but held his arms outright and gave Tom the hug of his life.

Tom smiled and while still hugging him said, "Charlie, it was great playing with you today. I am very sorry about what happened on ten. I wish I could have changed it."

Charlie suddenly released the hug and looked at Tom with a questioned look on his face. "What happened on ten? Did I make par?"

The End

www.ingramcontent.com/pod-product-compliance
Lightning Source LLC
LaVergne TN
LVHW051509080426

835509LV00017B/2005